Dirty Talk

How To Enhance Intimacy And Revitalize Your Romantic Connection: Utilizing Exemplary Expressions Of Desire To Heighten Your Relationship And Enrich Your Sexual Journey; Embracing Role Play To Ignite Passion In Your Partner

Peter Allison

TABLE OF CONTENT

Introduction 1
Unisex Phrases 13
Ensuring Readiness For Potential Inquiries 28
Avan 42
Promote And Foster An Environment That Encourages Individuals To Inquire And Engage In Candid, Open Dialogues 77
Inappropriate Discourse With Reserved Individuals 97
Dirty Conversations 102
Can The Practice Of Hypnosis Enhance One's Self-Assurance And Ease In Interpersonal Interactions With Women? 145
Understanding Emotional And Cultural Consent: Its Significance And Relevance 152
Middle Childhood 166

Introduction

Do you possess a basic understanding of how to engage in verbal communication with others? Approaching individuals at networking events, social gatherings, or in public settings can be perceived as intimidating in nature. However, it does not have to be this way! I must impart upon you uncomplicated techniques for engaging in conversations with individuals. All aspects fundamentally revolve around employing conversational techniques. Notwithstanding the absence of early instruction in this aptitude, I am keen to impart strategies for establishing swift and authentic connections with unfamiliar individuals.

Within the context of your professional responsibilities, you are likely to encounter a number of individuals, both affiliated with your organization and external to it. Having the ability to initiate conversations with individuals who are not familiar to you is a beneficial skill to possess when establishing new professional connections. Provide a comprehensive list of potential conversation starters to help you succeed in this particular domain. Within this publication, we present insights and examples of effective strategies for initiating a dialogue with an unfamiliar individual.

Some individuals possess the ability to engage in dialogue with any person, regardless of their familiarity or connection with them. Nevertheless, many individuals encounter difficulty when engaging in conversation with someone who is unfamiliar to them. This can be particularly distressing, particularly if you are afflicted with social anxiety disorder (SAD). Nevertheless, irrespective of any difficulty one may experience with engaging in social informal conversation, it is feasible to enhance one's conversational skills and cultivate an openness to engaging in dialogue with unfamiliar individuals. The most optimal approach to accomplish this goal is to engage in regular practice. Your initial aim should be to make a concise and straightforward statement that does not necessitate complexity. The purpose of initiating that initial comment is to establish a pathway for interaction, providing you with the opportunity to express something different upon receiving a response from the individual.

Additional information: Strategies for improving sexual receptiveness and exploration.

Enhanced or improved communication undoubtedly leads to a stronger bond and heightened intimacy within your relationship.

Nevertheless, honing your communication skills serves a broader purpose beyond merely improving your proficiency in engaging in discussions about intimate matters.

These are enduring proficiencies that will assist you in efficiently navigating your relationship on a daily basis. The greater your level of comfort in discussing matters such as sex and other subjects at any given time, the easier those significant discussions will appear.

To foster greater receptiveness and ease regarding this subject matter, it is necessary to establish a sense of normalcy through regular discussion. Do this by:

Reflecting on the cherished moments

While nestled in the coziness of the bed or the couch, engage in conversation about the instances wherein you both experienced mutually fulfilling intimate encounters, articulating the aspects that brought you immense pleasure during those noteworthy moments. Did the act, the physical contact, or the setting influence your attempt? Exhibit a penchant for exploration, and do not hesitate to vividly elucidate the minutiae to each other.

After identifying a particular aspect of an event that resonated with you, kindly express to your significant other your desire for a similar experience to be repeated. If you possess any insights pertaining to the occasion, do not hesitate to provide them.

Sexting

Amidst the hustle and bustle of a bustling day, a risqué message from your significant other possesses a profound effect beyond mere embarrassment. It elicits a sense of being desired, cherished, and filled with anticipation to return home and intimately disrobe your significant other.

Engaging in textual exchanges of a sexual nature can facilitate an increase in one's sexual receptiveness, as it enables individuals to discreetly communicate their longings and requirements to their partner, with the added advantage of having the liberty to provide explicit details.

For instance, one can send a message to their partner containing phrases like, "I eagerly anticipate the prospect of caressing your thigh and exploring every inch of your physique upon my arrival."

Engaging in the act of sending provocative messages can help maintain a stimulating dynamic in your relationship. It is recommended, however, to exercise moderation and refrain from inundating your partner's mobile device with an excessive number of explicit messages.

Discussing the explicit scenes

Have you encountered a situation in which you were engaged in viewing a program on HBO, and when a provocative scene unfolded, both you and your significant other were aroused? Well, you aren't alone.

Despite the existent social taboo surrounding discussions of such scenarios, let alone initiating a personal discussion based on them, there is no need for you to exhibit such discomfort.

In order to circumvent any potential discomfort observed while witnessing such portrayals on television, it is advisable to preemptively inform your partner of your intention to leverage such scenes for your mutual benefit.

Initiate a conversation when a scene is presented. For example, one could inquire their companion's opinion on whether they find it alluring when a woman engages in back-scratching while she and her partner are intimately engaged, presuming such a scenario aligns with the content being viewed.

Engage in jointly perusing a book dedicated to fostering interpersonal connections

Engage in the joint perusal of multiple literature pieces centered around fostering relationships, rather than limiting yourselves to a single tome. Engaging in a structured conversation may facilitate discussing matters pertaining to sexuality.

Cultivating your relationship extends beyond physical intimacy. Select a literary work comprising engaging and intellectually stimulating inquiries pertaining to subjects such as personal recollections from early years, intimate imaginings, and perspectives on interpersonal connections. The presence of a neutral intermediary facilitates a greater level of candor, wherein the book assumes the role of an objective third party.

Communicate during sex

During sexual intercourse, it is important to actively engage by providing both verbal and non-verbal communication to facilitate effective feedback, enabling your partner to ascertain their success in stimulating the desired areas.

When one experiences a strong sense of pleasure, it is appropriate to express it in the moment. Align your spine, rotate your gaze, attune yourself to the sensations within, and allow your body to convey its innate responses. Refrain from engaging in extensive discussions while engaging in sexual activity; focus on being present.

Be affectionate

Publicly display affection towards your partner. Embrace your partner as they engage in culinary activities; gently caress their neck with a kiss, and tenderly place a peck on their cheek as you both unwind for a peaceful evening.

Emotional attachment and physical intimacy are closely intertwined. As sexual frequency increases, the ability to express affection towards one's partner becomes enhanced, subsequently leading to an increased desire for sexual intimacy. The affectionate gestures shared in the kitchen might intensify and potentially result in intimate encounters on the kitchen counter.

On any occasion that affords the opportunity, demonstrate acts of affection towards your partner. To be more affectionate:

Engage in contact with your partner by embracing and expressing affection through kisses and hugs.

Please devote your complete focus and comprehension to your partner.

Maintain visual contact while exchanging thoughts.

Anticipate the needs of your partner and take proactive actions without necessitating their explicit requests.

Frequently communicate your profound affection for your partner and consistently articulate your emotions.

Assist your companion; this is a collaborative effort.

Engage in gaming activities, indulge in role-playing, and inject enthusiasm into the experience!

An effective approach to engage in lighthearted discussions regarding sex involves infusing an element of amusement, with numerous online games specifically designed to facilitate sexual communication.

Additionally, one may employ lighthearted activities such as 'Never have I Ever' and 'Truth or Dare' as methods of discerning the longings and preferences of one another. The main objective is to employ these games as a means to initiate more profound discussions.

In addition, one may engage in role-playing activities and arrange intimate evenings intermittently. You may choose to further explore and incorporate various intimate aids, such as introducing one or more items commonly known as sex toys. Please endeavor to diversify sexual experiences, moving away from traditional norms and exploring more varied and adventurous activities.

Suggestion: If one finds themselves experiencing discomfort when exposed to sexual terminology—possibly experiencing a reaction upon hearing terms such as cock, vagina, and so forth—an effective approach to alleviate this discomfort is to employ a psychological method known as flooding. This technique involves deliberately subjecting oneself to these words on a regular basis, gradually desensitizing oneself to their impact until they become less distressing. Position yourself in front of a mirror and recite the words as necessary. Speak those words silently to yourself; refrain from expressing them aloud to others.

Unisex Phrases

The explicit dialogue featured in this section is suitable for both sexes and can serve as an enjoyable method to invigorate your sexual experiences. If you are at an early stage, it is advisable to strive for the more moderate expressions. However, you have the liberty to incorporate your own verbiage or progress to the more intense phrases at your own pace.

You can utilize these various concepts for provocative discourse in order to devise personalized and alluring phrases. The key aspect lies in exhibiting ingenuity. Kindly utilize the following as a source of motivation.

Mild Dirty Talk
These expressions are straightforward to begin with and will assist in fostering a lighthearted ambiance conducive to intimate activities. When utilized effectively, they have the potential to

enhance your sensuality and simultaneously arouse your partner.

I want you.
You have the option to enhance this later by specifying the desired locations, instructions, or by incorporating a few expletives. For instance, "I intensely desire your presence in close proximity."

You're so hot/sexy.
There is no denying that a well-crafted, flattering remark has the potential to evoke feelings of attraction and arousal in someone.

I highly appreciate every aspect of your physique.
Express your admiration for your partner's physique by initiating the conversation with this statement, followed by a detailed account of the specific attributes you appreciate about each individual aspect.

Our compatibility is exceptional.
This sentiment is most ideally expressed upon initial intimacy, but is applicable at any juncture during the act of sexual intercourse.

It is imperative that you promptly remove those articles of clothing.
Want your lover naked? Tell them to strip. You have the option to either assist or observe in an entertaining performance involving the removal of clothing in a provocative manner.

You ignite my desire/arouse my interest.
Once more, it is universally appreciated to receive affirmation of one's ability to elicit a sexual response in their partner, thus making this statement advantageous to employ at the beginning stages of a relationship.

Your scent/appearance/flavor/tactility provokes an irresistible passion within me.

Select one perception and proceed with it. . . Alternatively, one may employ various iterations of praise within a single expression of admiration.

You are welcome to remain, however, the garments must be removed.
This is a straightforward proposition that will promptly lead to more pleasurable experiences.

It is imperative that we proceed with the recording of this particular moment.
When experiencing such synergy, it is imperative that this exceptional bond be documented on film, to be shared with the world (or exclusively between you both).

You possess exceptional intimate qualities that surpass any previous experiences I have had.
Elevate your lover to a position of admiration and ensure their profound worth is clearly communicated.

Stimulating your passion is something I thoroughly enjoy.
There should be no uncertainty that your purpose is to please. This is an enjoyable method to initiate intimate conversation with your significant other.

I greatly appreciate the fragrance/flavor/sensation that emanates from you.
In a similar vein as the previous statement, this allows you to elaborate on the perceptions your senses are discerning regarding the physical attributes of your beloved.

You elicit profound feelings of joy and contentment within me.
This expression holds applicability both in the context of foreplay and intimate moments, as well as following the completion of the act, in effectively conveying heartfelt sentiments concerning the actions of the individual involved.

Engage in playful banter with me until I am eagerly longing for it.
If one derives pleasure from playful banter, this approach serves as an ideal method for encouraging one's partner to engage in such behavior.

I expect you to be unclothed by the time I arrive at our residence.
Are you en route to your place of residence? Please ensure that you inform your partner of what they should anticipate upon your return. This is an exemplary text message to transmit.

Divine being, I am enamored by the sensation of your touch upon me.
These terms are exceptionally suitable for engaging in intimate conversation following sexual activity, or even during such moments... so get creative.

Our physical forms are ideally aligned for one another. They fit perfectly.
This can be employed in intimate situations, whether it be during a sexual

encounter or simply while cuddling, wherein her head fits snugly beneath your chin. It's romantic and sexy.

I intend to provide you with a pleasurable experience.
This phrase can be employed on various occasions, particularly when communicated via text or spoken with the intent of arranging a forthcoming encounter, pertaining to sexual activities.

The manner in which you walk/cook/talk greatly arouses my interest.
Irrespective of the activities your partner engages in, communicate to them that their actions arouse you. This approach effectively transforms a mundane task into an occasion of sensuality.

I earnestly desire to pursue this matter indefinitely.

Are you relishing the activities you engage in with your significant other? Inform them of the immense magnitude by expressing your aspiration to persevere indefinitely.

I could remain in this position of embrace with you indefinitely.
Provide an affirmative indication to your significant other that you are experiencing pleasure, even if you have not yet engaged in the actual event. This phrase can also be employed as intimate dialogue during moments of relaxation, subsequent to the occurrence.

I am greatly aroused by your presence/physique.
By communicating this, it typically imparts a sense of how erotically attractive you perceive your partner to be, while simultaneously kindling their desire.

You're amazing.
Who among us does not desire to be informed of their remarkable qualities?

This statement will be appreciated by individuals of both genders.

You taste like ____.
Incorporate delightful additions such as honey, vanilla, and similar ingredients. to evoke a feeling of enchantment or captivation in your romantic partner. This can also prove advantageous in instances where they exhibit a degree of reticence towards engaging in oral sexual activities.

You greatly vex me when you ____.
Select an activity that brings you pleasure when your significant other engages in it, and kindly motivate them to partake in it more frequently by utilizing this expression as a means to communicate your desires.

Your ____ is/are of exquisite beauty.
Select a preferred anatomical feature and effectively communicate your admiration thereof to your significant other. They will be deeply gratified, and it will further ignite their enthusiasm.

Uncertain about which anatomical region to prioritize? The visual appeal of one's eyes, lips, and neck can serve as an excellent point of departure.

Please remain silent and proceed to engage in a kiss with me.
Engaging in mutually stimulating directives can be arousing for both individuals, therefore, employ ingenuity to effectively communicate your desires to your partner.

I will be establishing the guidelines/taking charge this evening.
Although this may not be perceived as inappropriate, assuming authority can evoke a great deal of exhilaration. This expression also allows you to extend your actions through subsequent commands.

Please disregard all arrangements made for this evening. Tonight you're mine.

Assume control and strategically devise plans to ignite an invigorating atmosphere through the utilization of explicit discourse.

As you wish.
Is there anyone who wouldn't appreciate the opportunity to have a genie fulfill their every desire? Although you may not possess magical powers like a genie, you can undeniably bring immense delight to your partner by attentively fulfilling their desires.

You have a profound positive impact on my emotional state.
Your romantic partner will make diligent efforts to enhance your well-being upon learning of this.

You are truly exceptional, my dear.
This is an elegant and straightforward sentence that will undoubtedly stir their enthusiasm. Moreover, they will strive to enhance their previous achievements.

Please engage in intimate relations with me. I need you.
Engaging in intimate relations is a more refined approach to discussing sexual activity and may instill a greater sense of comfort if one is new to explicit language.

How have I been fortunate enough to have such good fortune?
Elevate the praise for your partner by articulating the remarkable qualities that encompass their entire being, encompassing their captivating gaze and alluring attributes.

Oh, my goodness, that sensation is incredibly pleasurable!
On occasion, maintaining a state of simplicity suffices. It is advisable to effectively communicate your preferences to your partner, as they will be inclined to prioritize those actions that bring you pleasure.

You're going to make me reach climax already.
There is no better expression of attraction and desire than conveying to your partner that they can bring you to climax quickly.

That is excellent, continue with your efforts.
Like what they're doing? Then inform them accordingly in order to encourage perseverance.

Tell me you're mine.
In the event that you discover an affinity for engaging in explicit conversation, whilst your partner exhibits timidity, you may instruct them on the preferred language to utilize.

I desire to thoroughly examine every intricate detail of your physique.
Articulate the statement before commencing the action for utmost impact. Use lips, fingers, etc. to engage in

the pursuit of discovery while maintaining an alluring ambiance.

I find it quite challenging to endure the absence of physical contact with you.
If one is unable to spend time together intermittently, employing this expression will intensify the other person's desire for oneself to an even greater extent.

I had never realized the depths of my longing for someone until now.
If your significant other is evoking new emotions within you, do not hesitate to express it to them, allowing them to bask in the feeling of uniqueness.

Your lips are irresistible.
While initiating by acknowledging their lips may be a suitable course of action, it is vital to recognize that there are several other captivating features on the body. Hence, it is imperative to have the confidence to explore and discuss those as well.

Are you aware of the impact your actions have upon me?
If they are unaware of the impact they have on you, it is appropriate to communicate your feelings to them. . . going into great detail.

I am willing to comply with your requests. Kindly provide me with the necessary details regarding the time and location.
The exclusive opportunity to have your undivided attention, along with the authority to dictate how they should care for their body, is a privilege that most romantic partners will deeply value. And make the most of.

Ensuring Readiness For Potential Inquiries

Undoubtedly, your daughter will undoubtedly have inquiries or additional matters of interest. She may also exhibit reluctance to express her thoughts as she lacks certainty regarding the appropriate manner to do so. Once more, provide her with assurance that she can approach you with any inquiry and that you will respond to her questions to the best of your ability. In order to assist you in your preparation, the following questions can be anticipated.

Potential Inquiries Your Daughter May Pose:

- What is the reason behind the development of my breasts? What is the reason behind the increase in size of my hips?

The period of puberty readies the human body for the subsequent phase of life, known as adulthood. Each young woman will undergo physical changes characterized by an increase in breast size and widening of the hips, serving as a biological preparation for the role of motherhood.

• What is the reason for the disparity in size between my breasts and those of other girls?
Each girl's physical maturation is distinct, with some undergoing earlier breast and hip development, while others may experience their physical changes at a delayed rate. An individual's physique, encompassing the development of breast size, is genetically determined. Similar to the unique attributes of one's hair or eye color, this will vary among each individual girl.

• I am curious as to why a female student in my class does not experience menstruation.

It is possible that she is maturing at a slower pace. She will imminently experience menstruation, as it is an inevitable part of the pubescent development that all females undergo.

• May I inquire as to the reason for the significant increase in height of my fellow classmate compared to my own stature?

A considerable number of adolescents experience growth spurts, with certain individuals progressing at an earlier pace than others. Furthermore, the expression of specific genetic traits significantly influences the ultimate height that an individual can attain.

• Could you please provide an explanation of the concept of masturbation? Is it bad? Can I do it?

Masturbation is an inherent physiological response aimed at alleviating sexual tension. Sexual tension can also be deflected or channeled into alternative activities such as engaging in sports or pursuing hobbies. Deciding whether to permit a child to engage in masturbation is an individual choice that should be influenced by your personal values and inclinations. Please instruct your child on the importance of carrying out such actions in a discreet manner. Like many other things, developing an addiction to it is detrimental to one's wellbeing.

- What is the cause behind the sensation of tingling that I experience internally when encountering the young man I am fond of?

The endocrine system within the human body has the capability to elicit a myriad of emotions and sensations. Adolescents frequently develop strong infatuations and may encounter physiological stimulation akin to the heightened anticipation one experiences before attending a highly anticipated concert or indulging in a cherished gastronomic delight. It is crucial to engage in thoughtful deliberation prior to responding or making decisions, ensuring that emotions are contemplated through cognitive processes rather than relying solely on intuitive or visceral responses.

May I inquire about the permissibility of removing my pubic hair?
Yes. Similar to the strands of hair adorning your scalp or other regions of the body, it is deemed acceptable to trim or groom one's pubic hair. This signifies that there are no adverse health ramifications associated with shaving, although individual preferences or religious convictions may differ. Greater emphasis should be placed on upholding and practicing proper hygiene, while exercising caution in doing so.

Your offspring might astound you with the inquiries she wishes to pose. Don't be ruffled, though. Please bear in mind that you, too, experienced adolescence at one point in your life. You possess a comprehensive understanding of her emotions and possess personal knowledge about the process of adolescence. In case you experience some degree of being overburdened when she catches you off guard with her inquiries, simply recall your own state during that stage of your life. In the event that you find yourself unable to provide a conventional response to a question, it would be advisable to offer her a reply grounded in personal anecdotal evidence. She will establish a stronger connection with you if she is aware that you have experienced identical circumstances to the ones she is presently facing.

Chapter 3 – The Female Leader

Please make way - it is now my turn to assume control.

I intend to secure your hands to the headboard of the bed.

Given that typically, there are solely two mutually consenting adults present in the bedroom, one of these individuals must take the initiative. Frequently, this tends to be rather weak following the prolonged duration of a relationship. He inquires about her current disposition, to which she responds affirmatively or negatively, and subsequently engages in intimate activity; nonetheless, there exists possibilities to enliven this experience. It is essential for individuals to comprehend that initiating sexual activities centers around comprehending one's partner's preferences and skillfully stimulating their desires to cultivate interest.

Requesting what one desires

For example, in the event that a woman desires sexual intimacy, why is it not acceptable for her to prompt her partner to lie on his back, encourage him to remove any clothing, and convey her readiness and willingness? Addressing him in a commanding manner such as, 'I shall assume charge now,' may elicit arousal and captivate his attention. Women are inclined to exhibit a reduced propensity for positively reacting to utterances perceived as inappropriate and discourteous. It may give them a sense of diminished value, even though considering the roles both individuals assume within the confines of the intimate space, it is reasonable to argue that their true selves, which may not meet societal norms, are not deemed improper within that setting. It entails assuming a role for the purpose of deriving sexual gratification. Hence, words that would typically deviate from one's usual discourse may be deemed appropriate as long as both parties are aware of their impending utterance.

She might assertively request the maximum effort from him, as she leans forward with her chest and positions herself on top of him. That is deemed acceptable and encouraging, as opposed to being perceived as demeaning and shocking. The crux of the matter lies in your ability to assess the situation and employ suitable language corresponding to its nature. Intimate relations involve more than mere physical interactions; effective communication during these exchanges can significantly enhance the passion and allure of the experience. On certain occasions, merely producing sounds in the appropriate locations falls short of the intended outcome. If he accurately stimulates the Grafenberg spot, there is no issue with expressing to the individual that they have successfully located it. "Indeed, my dear, indeed." "That is exquisite!" informs him of his accurate performance, which inevitably serves as an encouragement for him to continue exhibiting such favorable conduct.

Similarly, a gentleman can employ comparable forms of provocative discourse and playful banter to motivate and exhilarate his partner in a comparable manner. I desire that you envelop me within the realm of your lips," expresses his preferences clearly and artfully. Such explicit communication serves as a vital conduit, for without it, one might stumble blindly, yearning for an outcome that may ultimately elude them, leading to profound disappointment. If he is accustomed to engaging in sexual activities in a dimly lit environment, gently leaning over his body and switching on the light, accompanied by the phrase, "I desire to witness your heightened arousal, rather than obscure it with darkness," effectively conveys your affection for his physique, which is undeniably quite passionate. Many males possess desires to engage in sexual intercourse with the lights illuminated, and when incorporating suggestive language, their arousal is further heightened.

He can provide her with encouragement by switching on the light. Her physique arouses me deeply and evokes strong physical responses, which could potentially be the motivation she requires. If a female individual carries a slight excess weight, it is conceivable that she is mindful of the matter. Nevertheless, it might actually serve as a source of attraction for the male individual. Approach me, young lady, so that I may behold the splendor of your bosom. Although it may appear unremarkable, it possesses a certain allure. It serves to affirm her identity and bolster her self-assurance.

The lady occasionally requires assuming a leadership role. Alternatively, sex can begin to feel somewhat mechanized or devoid of emotional connection. She may strategically employ the phrase, 'Please stimulate this area,' to her advantage, while also benefiting him by aiding him in locating the G spot and alleviating any instances of clumsiness. The predicament lies in the fact that there exists a societal inclination for women to adhere to prescribed behavioral patterns, while men are expected to consistently embody chivalrous qualities. Nevertheless, societal norms hold no significance within the confines of the bedroom. If a woman desires something, there is no impropriety in asserting her rights to it and deriving satisfaction upon its accomplishment.

Engaging in provocative language to provoke his arousal.

As an engaging gesture, the act of teasing can involve delaying his climax through communication such as, "Hold on, I have strategic intentions for your pleasure!" and guiding him into a position where the woman assumes dominance. This can be succeeded by engaging in a leisurely lovemaking experience or even engaging in oral stimulation until the point just prior to his climax, ensuring that his penis is inserted into her only when she desires it, as opposed to solely relying on his initiative. "I will cause you discomfort!" might be his reply, and he could indeed deliver on that statement, subsequently suggesting to alleviate the pain when she expresses her dissatisfaction with the resulting inflammation.

Women who assume control within the realm of intimacy effectively convey a sense of assertiveness and provide their partners with the perception that they possess a clear understanding of their desires. Additionally, this dynamic offers an opportunity for men to delve into their own sexual exploration. The range of vocabulary should be expanded beyond mere repetition of the term "more" since doing so enhances the enjoyment of sexual activities and allows her to confidently express her desire for complete satisfaction, thus intensifying the overall experience.

One should not presume that a woman must conform to societal expectations of being tender and feminine in the realm of intimacy, unless, of course, that is the particular inclination that excites her partner. Using the appropriate language to stimulate his arousal, she has the ability to assume various roles such as a partner of authority, a provocateur, or a key catalyst during the peak of his pleasure. It is deemed appropriate and could potentially serve as the determining factor in ensuring that she attains an equal level of gratification as he does.

Good sir, please kindly recline and face the challenge with fortitude. "I shall assume command this evening!" as you assertively guide your partner onto the bed and begin removing your garments, is a bold declaration that captivates a man's attention and ignites intense desire. Witnessing a woman who confidently pursues her desires with unwavering determination is an immensely arousing experience for any man. Why not demonstrate your proficiency with the use of your vibrator? Engage in close proximity in order for him to observe the specific factors that elicit a response from your G spot, as well as comprehend the auditory cues accompanying said response. He might even derive great amusement from it and occasionally jokingly jest with you, in order to evoke a highly receptive reaction.

Avan

FUCK. HE WAS the sheriff? Was I placed under arrest?

Why didn't he mention this sooner? I had been engaged in conversation with him in a foolish manner, entirely oblivious to the fact that he had intentions of incarcerating me.

Undoubtedly, a correctional facility would not be able to confine me. I had recently undergone a vicious attack by a wild creature, relied on soliciting rides from individuals, and subsequently experienced pursuit by a property owner armed with a firearm.

Among the various unfortunate circumstances, this is the most unfortunate. An apprehension would be detrimental to my application for admission to the bar association. The majority of states desired for their legal practitioners to possess upright character and lack any criminal record.

This arrest, in particular, was of significant consequence. It constituted an apprehension on charges of unauthorized intrusion. Might he also consider bringing charges of theft against me?

Surely not.

He had provided significant assistance by tending to the wound on my abdomen.

Despite his ongoing denial of being the person in question.

I had desired to place my trust in him. Every fiber of my being was adamantly suggesting that I should. But now? I wasn't so sure.

He maintained his outstretched hand in my direction, displaying an apparent intention to offer assistance with my standing. Please refrain from making physical contact with me. Although I intended to cooperate, I had no intention of doing so in a cordial manner.

I was aware of the imprudence of the situation, yet I couldn't suppress a sense of slight betrayal. I had believed that there existed a certain connection or bond between the two of us. The smile he exhibited upon hearing my name led me to believe that it held significance.

I rose to a standing position at a deliberate pace. Although my skin continued to experience discomfort, there was no reoccurrence of bleeding. I extended my arms outward, yet he refrained from placing handcuffs upon me.

If you are willing to cooperate, there won't be a necessity for those.

I let out an exasperated sigh, yet refrained from engaging in any dispute.

"May I inquire about your current state of well-being?" he inquired.

I am adequately well for the time being. In the unlikely eventuality of any personal affliction, I would prefer not to divulge the information to him.

Please inform me in case you experience any discomfort. We will pay a visit to the hospital.

I huffed. Oh, I assumed my alleged criminality was deemed significant enough to warrant immediate transportation to the correctional facility.

He demonstrated an overt display of dismissiveness by audibly rotating his eyes in a upward, circular motion. We are committed to providing medical assistance to all individuals without exception.

Are the taxpayers aware of your engagement in arbitrary detentions?

"The citizens happen to express approval of the job I am performing," he stated.

And by what means do you possess such knowledge?

Given that I have been chosen as the elected representative on four separate occasions.

I laughed. He displayed a great deal of arrogance and took pride in his own accomplishments. What is the assurance that you do not coerce or intimidate them into casting their votes in your favor?

It is likely that their voting decision was influenced by their perception of his physical attractiveness. He would appear highly presentable and distinguished in attire consistent with a formal dress code.

At that juncture, he approached me closely. "I\\\'m not a bully."

My cardiac frequency increased, accompanied by a pleasant sensation of butterflies in my abdomen. I did not perceive any sense of threat to my physical well-being. There was an alternative situation unfolding, and I possessed complete awareness of its true nature.

I experienced it while situated on the mountainside, at the moment of my rescue by him.

I was turned on.

Aroused.

That is precisely what the sensation entailed.

That had a modicum of coherence. But now? Was I unaware of a preference or inclination I possessed? Had I harbored a long-standing desire to be apprehended by a law enforcement officer, and is this encounter the realization of my clandestine fetish?

That made no sense.

And the sensation of my stimulation seemed to be distinct. Although my arousal was evident, I also experienced a profound discomfort within me.

I have always had a preference for engaging in sexual relations. That was nothing new. However, this discomfort was unfamiliar. I had a strong desire to be fulfilled promptly.

Was his cock big? I was seeking to ascertain.

Not going to happen.

He graciously assisted me into the vehicle by opening the car door.

Having taken my place within the confines of his vehicle, feeling a measure of security, my mind was no longer solely occupied with thoughts of apprehension and the imminent prospect of incarceration.

I could contemplate upon the information he had shared, specifically his denial of undergoing a transformation into a wolf.

At first glance, it would be logical to place belief in his words. However, my intuition unequivocally affirmed the accuracy of my position. He underwent a metamorphosis and assumed the form of a lupine creature. I had observed the event take place. I did experience a loss of blood. However, I was not experiencing any delusions.

I had also observed a palpable sense of fear in his eyes upon my confrontation regarding the wolf. He had not anticipated my awareness of his capability for transformation, and it was evidently apparent that he was unaccustomed to being challenged with inquiries.

I had reached the conclusion that it would be imprudent for me to persist in the idea that he was a wolf, hence requiring me to make slight workforce reductions. There is a possibility that the situation carried some level of danger, although my gut instinct assured me of his non-threatening nature.

Perhaps it was intended for him to refrain from disclosing this information. Might that be the reason for which he was apprehending me? In order to prevent disseminating the information?

However, who would place trust in my words?

No one. That\\\'s who. Particularly upon learning about the incident involving my encounter with coyotes, and his subsequent act of rescue. Any assessment or evaluation I made subsequent to experiencing such distressing trauma would be subject to scrutiny.

Indeed, was he veritably regarded as the esteemed sheriff of the town? In such a scenario, I would potentially become a source of concern if I were to engage in the act of making unfounded allegations against him. They would perceive me as being delusional or possibly engaging in stalking behavior.

Given the circumstances, it was difficult for me to dwell on the thought, but it was undeniable that he possessed exceptional physical attractiveness. He possessed the characteristics that would attract the attention of an unstable individual, further reinforcing the necessity for me to maintain silence.

Nonetheless, refraining from expressing my thoughts was simply not innate to my character. "I promise to maintain utmost confidentiality," I assured.

"What is it that you would like to disclose?" he inquired.

The veracity pertaining to your true identity.

I was observing him intently, and true to my observations, his entire physique convulsed upon uttering the words. It wasn\\\'t much. He effectively concealed it. However, the response remained present.

What is the veracity concerning my identity? I\\\'m a sheriff."

Right. I was onto something. I gazed intently through the window. I lacked familiarity with the town, yet it appeared that we were proceeding in a direction contrary to the central area, where one would expect to find a correctional facility. It appears that our current trajectory is leading us deeper into rural areas.

"Where are we going?"

He didn\\\'t answer. However, he managed to decelerate the vehicle.

"May I inquire, Sheriff, as to the precise destination you are bringing me to?" I inquired. It is within my entitlement to be informed.

Upon briefly diverting his gaze towards me, he began to speak. I am aware that our initial interactions have been less than smooth. And that\\\'s my fault. However, it is imperative that you place your trust in me.

What reasons do you provide for me to place my trust in you?

Due to the existence of concepts that may elude your comprehension.

That much was obvious. "So tell me."

The car slowed down. However, rather than heading towards the bustling city center or the heart of a quaint town, our route veered onto a unpaved gravel road.

A sensation of unease enveloped me, causing my skin to tingle. "Sheriff. I would like to ascertain our destination. This facility does not function as a correctional institution."

He sighed. "No. It's not."

I reached for the door handle. Whilst I cannot claim to be explicitly afraid of him, it is worth noting that he had indeed deceived me. Over and over. I forcefully pulled the door handle. If it were possible for me to safely exit the vehicle, it would greatly improve my situation.

We were encircled by trees from either direction. There was, in any event, a possibility that I could flee and seek refuge in the surrounding forest.

As I gently ajar the door, his arm swiftly extended and seized my wrist. He exerted minimal force, yet his grasp wielded sufficient strength to immobilize me. He sternly warned against exiting the vehicle hastily.

I refuse to remain seated in this position and allow you to transport me to an undisclosed destination.

I regret to inform you that I am unable to accompany you to an undisclosed destination.

"May I inquire as to where you are intending to escort me?" I firmly requested.

"To my house."

"Your house? In what manner can I be apprehended within the confines of your residence? Do not assert that this locality is so lacking in modernity that you manage mug shots from the comfort of your own residence. My goodness. What if he did not possess the occupation of a sheriff? In contemporary times, obtaining a uniform has become relatively accessible to the general populace.

"No," he decelerated the vehicle further. I hereby declare that I am not actually detaining or apprehending you.

This exceeded my initial expectations by a significant margin. In light of the fact that he had indeed abducted me, incarceration would have constituted a more suitable measure in this circumstance.

HOW TO APPROACH CHILDREN ABOUT SEX FROM INFANCY TO AGE TWO.

Whilst it may appear daunting to acquaint your child with the anatomically accurate terminology for their genitalia, it is essential to adopt a formal approach and treat those terms with the same level of casualness as you would use words such as "arm" or "ankle," refraining from undue association of gender with sexual biology.

Disregard the belief that all males possess penises and all females possess vaginas, to provide an example. Please utilize the phrases "Individuals with female reproductive anatomy" or "Individuals with male reproductive anatomy" in place of the previous statement. By exercising caution in your choice of language today, you lay the groundwork for future discussions on gender identities and roles that are more straightforward.

Parents are advised to commence the imparting of knowledge to their children regarding the appropriate context and circumstances in which they may engage in self-exploration of their bodies at the age of two. Take the opportunity to clarify that engaging with our genitalia is a private matter limited to the confines of our bedrooms, if your child demonstrates a tendency towards this behavior, which is considered quite typical. Avoid instilling a sense of guilt in your child through excessive gentleness in your explanation.

How to Approach Conversations on Human Reproduction with Children Aged 2-5

Understanding boundaries and discerning what is acceptable in terms of physical contact, both in terms of initiating it or receiving it, is a significant subject for individuals in this particular stage of development. It is imperative for even young children to acquire the habit of seeking permission prior to making physical contact with another individual. A deeper understanding of consent can be cultivated by engaging in educational activities, interactive games involving physical contact, such as gentle tickling, and establishing personal boundaries whereby communicating explicit instructions to a child about the appropriateness of sitting on one's lap can be helpful.

Asserting the principle that children possess autonomy over their own bodies further enhances their safety. Notwithstanding the possibility of omitting explicit details, it is crucial to use this opportunity to instill in your child the principle of never engaging in discussions or physical contact concerning their private body parts. It is of utmost importance to stress that irrespective of any past concealment, your children have the liberty to approach you at any given moment with regards to any instances of misconduct.

Children may exhibit curiosity towards one another's physical aspects during this developmental stage. It is imperative to acknowledge this inquisitiveness and leverage it as a launching pad for discussing your family's customs and principles. Provide a comprehensive elucidation to them regarding the circumstances in which it is deemed appropriate to be fully exposed. In the event that you observe your children engaging in imaginative play as doctors, it is advised to maintain your composure. On the contrary, it is important to address the notion that the genitalia of others are highly personal and confidential areas of the body, which should be respected and not subject to unauthorized physical contact.

At this stage of development, your child may begin to question the process by which infants are conceived. Based on your perception of your young child's comprehension level, you have the flexibility to provide an extensive or limited amount of information. If your child expresses further curiosity, you may explain that adults engage in a process where their bodies unite to combine the sperm and the egg, resulting in the creation of a child like you. Alternatively, they may acquire the sperm or egg from a third party. It's acceptable to explain to your child certain specifics, such as how the sperm and egg combine.

Please be mindful to refrain from telling untruths. It is imperative to actively engage in asking those subsequent inquiries instead of simply refusing to broach certain subjects.

Informing children of their own birth story provides an opportunity to tailor the information to the specific circumstances of your family, all the while initiating a discussion on the process of infant creation. Please keep in mind that families can be formed in various ways, and your child's birth narrative is just one among them.

It is of paramount importance to educate children within this age group about the multitude of approaches to forming families and cultivating relationships. Your children will undoubtedly become aware of this phenomenon if they are affiliated with non-conventional family structures or engage extensively in their company.

Nevertheless, should that not be the case, ensure you possess a selection of superb literary works that do not exclusively center around nuclear, heterosexual households.

Moreover, employ inclusive language in your everyday communication. Modify the phrase "Welcome, boys and girls" to alternatives such as "Welcome, children" or "Welcome, young ones," for example. This subtle alteration impart to children the concept that gender is not confined to binary categorizations, thus promoting a more inclusive understanding.

Strategies for Addressing the Topic of Human Reproduction with Children Ages 6-8

Despite the fact that your child will not be granted unsupervised access to the internet for a few more years, it remains imperative to initiate discussions with them at present regarding the methods by which they can navigate digital environments securely. Ensure that your child possesses an understanding of the regulations pertaining to engaging in conversation with unfamiliar individuals, sharing images on the internet, and the appropriate course of action to take if encountering any situation causing discomfort.

While it may not be necessary to provide children with explicit explanations about pornography from the start, it is important to be prepared for the possibility of them encountering it. Elucidate in a composed manner that said websites pertain to the behavior of mature individuals. While it is not imperative to depict pornography as morally reprehensible, it is advised to acknowledge that these websites are strictly intended for adult viewership.

Considering that the majority of children commence the process of self-awareness and self-exploration around the age of eight, this presents an opportune moment to discuss the subject of masturbation. Please remember to discuss the importance of proper hygiene, emphasizing its commonplace nature and the need for individuals to address it in the privacy of their personal spaces.

At this stage of development, it is appropriate to engage in more explicit conversations with children regarding the topic of sexual assault. Children must be made cognizant of this unfortunate reality in order to either safeguard themselves or aid a comrade who may be experiencing abuse. The extent of this conversation will ultimately be determined by your child. I recommend commencing your approach by emphasizing the foundational principles, such as the significance of only engaging with them with explicit permission. Subsequently, endeavor to ascertain their comprehension and emotional response through a follow-up interaction several days later.

It may be advisable to delay discussing this matter until your child reaches a more mature age if they display signs of anger.

At this juncture, it may be appropriate to impart upon children a comprehensive understanding of the fundamental mechanisms pertaining to human reproduction. It is essential to highlight that there is no inherent issue with introducing this information to your child at an early stage, provided they demonstrate readiness, or deferring its introduction slightly if you assess that they may not comprehend it.

Engaging in discourse surrounding sexuality and the physiological changes associated with puberty can be regarded as interrelated topics. This can be an uncomplicated discourse regarding the transformations that occur in the human physique during early childhood, typically around the age of six. One could, for example, juxtapose childhood photographs of them with recent portraits. The comprehensive conversation regarding puberty should be rescheduled to occur shortly before your child or individuals within her social circle start encountering its effects. Alternatively, it may convey the impression that you are engaging in conversation about an extraterrestrial realm.

The onset of puberty in females typically occurs between the ages of nine and eleven in individuals possessing female reproductive anatomy. For those individuals, the development of breast buds, a process that generally commences prior to the age of 10, is an essential indicator that this transition is occurring.

In subsequent years, commonly at approximately 12 years of age (although earlier occurrences are not uncommon), the onset of menstruation arises. Puberty typically initiates in individuals with male genitalia around the age of 10, marked by the initial manifestation of pubic hair growth as the most observable indication.

I recommend engaging in the activity of reading a well-written literary material alongside your child, focused on the topic of puberty. This will enable both of you to acquire knowledge about the scientific intricacies associated with this phase of life. Such literature would provide valuable insights into the distinctions between testosterone and estrogen, as well as elucidate the causes and mechanisms underlying bodily transformations such as hair growth, genital development, voice modulation, and so forth. Facilitate a discourse that includes everyone. Females are not granted a lesson, while males are also not granted a lesson. Children ought to receive instruction regarding alternate forms of human anatomy in addition to their own.

The ramifications of this transition ought to be a matter of ongoing discourse, despite the fact that the intricacies of puberty's mechanisms may only be deliberated upon on a single occasion.

It is equally significant for children of this age to acquire knowledge regarding the diverse manifestations of gender. Prior to engaging with the topic, conduct thorough research if it is one which you have been consciously evading. I strongly recommend discussing the point that an individual's gender cannot be ascertained based on their genitalia.

The Scientific Explanation behind the Erotic Stimulation of Verbalized Obscenities

When considering sexual arousal, the minds of the majority of individuals promptly tend to focus on their reproductive organs. Am I right? You envisage all the sensory experiences linked to arousal. The sensation of tingling, warmth, and eager anticipation associated with the prospect of a loving caress or contact with one's erogenous areas. For the majority of individuals, engaging in sexual intercourse entails a corporeal experience accompanied by profound sensations and emotions. It is imperative for our purposes to comprehend that sexual arousal constitutes an entirely distinct phenomenon.

Sexual stimulation typically occurs prior to engaging in sexual intercourse. It initiates within the confines of one's mind before extending to the realm of physical intimacy. This element contributes to the immense pleasure and stimulation that dirty talk evokes. Engaging in risqué conversation with your partner can initiate a strong physical attraction towards you well before any intimate encounters take place. Engaging in explicit conversation stimulates arousal in the psyche, thereby amplifying physical sensations. Fostering a more profound physical and emotional bond. This process initiates within the cranial region.

Various regions of the brain that govern phenomena such as sexual motivation and stimulation. Engaging in provocative discourse with your partner activates specific regions of the cerebral cortex that incite sexual arousal. Engaging in suggestive discourse fulfills our yearning for interpersonal connection and satiates our inclination towards physical intimacy.

As a result of this, engaging in explicit communication during intimate moments fosters a multidimensional sexual encounter that stimulates various cognitive processes in the brain. This notion of sexuality through insinuation can prolong the sensation of arousal beyond mere tactile stimulation. The human brain exhibits a high susceptibility to suggestion. Occasionally, the concept or idea of a thing can possess an equal potency to the tangible manifestation itself. This is partially why engaged in explicit verbal expressions can effectively excite individuals.

The Rationale Behind the Pleasurable Sensations of Erotic Communication

Engaging in explicit language stimulates certain areas of the brain simultaneously with the physiological arousal of the body.

Verbal obscenities elicit neural response in the identical regions of the brain associated with offensive language. This implies that the more explicit and provocative the explicit language is, the greater the potential for excitement and arousal.

Individuals who derive pleasure from submissiveness frequently find enjoyment in engaging in explicit communication due to its relation to the experience of fear within the brain. The area of the brain associated with fear is intricately interconnected with feelings of pleasure and exhilaration. This inherent association can elicit significant intellectual arousal.

Vocalizations such as moans, screams, and whispers elicit neural responses within the auditory cortex. This establishes a direct link to arousing your partner's senses.

Engaging in provocative conversation can serve as a pathway to exploring one's fantasies. This can still evoke excitement, regardless of whether you or your partner lack the inclination to enact these fantasies in a genuine setting. The sensitive nature of addressing such matters heightens stimulation. The mind visualizes the prohibited actions and triggers physical sensations within the body.

Research suggests that engaging in open discourse regarding matters of intimacy and sexual experiences positively contributes to overall relationship contentment among partners.

Certain individuals are capable of attaining orgasm solely through the act of indulging in explicit verbal communication.

The Mentality of Virtue and Vice

You might be familiar with the concept of the "ideal woman" or the "virtuous woman" phenomenon. Many men fantasize about having a woman who initially embodies a pleasant and charming persona like the girl residing nearby, but later transforms into a sexually adventurous individual within the confines of the bedroom. Enthusiastically committed to fulfilling the man's every request.

Engaging in explicit language facilitates a constructive and empowering avenue for women to delve into these societal roles. During explicit conversations, women have the ability to distance themselves from their more traditional or reserved aspects. They derive pleasure from being referred to using derogatory language or engaging in consensual bondage. Actions that would typically be deemed inappropriate in a non-intimate setting can now induce stimulation and enjoyment.

It is ultimately within your prerogative as a woman to determine the extent to which boundaries should not be crossed. Women have the capacity to derive a sense of empowerment from their sexual desires, without the need to harbor feelings of shame or guilt concerning them. Engaging in erotic communication serves as a pathway to the attainment of personal empowerment. A means of exchanging thoughts and exploring pleasurable experiences within a nurturing sexual setting.

Engaging in erotic dialogue can serve as an effective means for couples to explore concepts of power dynamics, such as dominance and submission. If you tend to assert more authority in your professional endeavors, you may find the notion of assuming a submissive role for an evening appealing, or alternatively, if you generally adopt a submissive approach, you might entertain the idea of temporarily embracing a dominant role. Engaging in explicit conversations opens up boundless avenues for exploring novel roles and fantasies.

Engaging in explicit communication involves articulating your desires and preferences to augment the quality of your intimate encounters. In order for explicit communication to yield profound results, it must be approached as a collaborative endeavor. Both yourself and your significant other are expected to engage in a manner that is both supportive and encouraging.

Occasionally, the use of explicit language can elicit discomfort or come across as humorous. Please be mindful that it is permissible to express humor and engage in light-hearted behavior. Engaging in explicit discourse is intended to be entertaining. It is imperative for both you and your partner to ensure comfort and enjoyment in order to prevent the onset of negative emotions such as resentment or insecurity.

Promote And Foster An Environment That Encourages Individuals To Inquire And Engage In Candid, Open Dialogues.

When observing a heightened curiosity towards sexuality in your child, it is imperative to foster an environment that encourages inquiry and facilitates sincere and transparent discussions with them. As per extensive studies, sexual content pervades various forms of media, particularly when one has access to cable television, the internet, or other media platforms.

There is no alternative method to ensure your comfort, knowledge, and sense of safety regarding matters pertaining to sexuality than engaging in open and unrestricted discussions on the topic. You will gain an understanding of the importance of fostering an environment that promotes curiosity and encourages your young ones to inquire and participate in transparent and sincere discussions. Rest assured that by employing this approach, your child will develop a comprehensive understanding of the practical implications associated with human sexuality.

The Significance of Engaging in Transparent and Sincere Dialogues with Your Offspring.

It is incumbent upon you, as a parent, to engage in open and transparent conversations about sexuality with your child. Sexual apprehension may be alleviated through open and truthful communication between parents and their children.

The objective of engaging in open and candid conversations regarding sexual matters with one's child is centered on the exploration and exchange of viewpoints relating to personal inclinations and preferences. Engaging in open and candid conversations about sex with your child will greatly influence their life in a positive manner.

Engaging in constructive, transparent, and candid dialogues concerning sexuality can greatly aid your child in equipping themselves for potential eventualities.

When your child inquires about sex, it is imperative that you furnish them with accurate information and verified facts that are satisfactory to them.

It is imperative that you additionally undertake thorough research on your own accord to ensure you are equipping your child with the specific information they seek.

CHAPTER SIX

Conduct an inquiry into the curriculum being taught at the child's educational institution.

In the present era, virtually all institutions and educational establishments offer a comprehensive sexual education curriculum for their students. As an accountable guardian, it is essential for you to remain knowledgeable about the educational content being imparted to your child, particularly within the confines of their classroom.

Certain individuals experience unease and bewilderment upon encountering the term 'sex.' It is crucial to investigate the curriculum being employed in your child's classroom, particularly when you notice that they are facing such circumstances, especially within an educational institution.

The Veracity Regarding Academically Acquired Educational Resources
The prevailing practice adopted by the majority of educational institutions entails the utilization of sex education literature that can conveniently be procured both commercially and via digital platforms. The majority of sexual education literature comprises intricate guidelines that can significantly aid individuals in acquiring comprehensive understanding of sexual matters.

Expanding your child's knowledge and understanding of human sexuality is one of the primary motivations behind the inclusion of sex education classes in various educational institutions.

The majority of sex education literature recommends initiating conversations about sex with your child prior to the manifestation of any sexual behaviors.

Consequently, sexual education classes are meticulously designed and implemented to provide your child with discernment and information that can be utilized in the imminent future, particularly when they are prepared to navigate the practical aspects of the realm of sexuality.

Rest assured that through the implementation of sex education programs and courses offered at educational institutions, your child will have access to invaluable knowledge and guidance pertaining to sexual orientation, safe sexual practices, and abstinence.

Furthermore, there are sexual health services available to provide assistance to your adolescent in addressing any inquiries related to sexuality. Due to the accessibility of these sexual health services, your child will have the opportunity to acquire comprehensive knowledge about sexuality in an environment that ensures their safety and comfort.

The potential consequences of avoiding discussions about sexual education and relationships.

It is imperative that you possess a thorough understanding and appreciation of the extensive breadth of knowledge and intricacies surrounding the topic of sex, so as to avert any potential repercussions during discussions pertaining to this subject matter.

Experiencing initial discomfort and unease is a common response when engaging in conversations pertaining to sexuality with your child.

Nevertheless, it is crucial to remember that engaging in conversations about human sexuality with your child during their early years can yield notable advantages, such as mitigating the risks of unintended pregnancies and establishing the groundwork for a secure future for them.

It is highly recommended that you engage in open and constructive discussions with your child regarding topics related to their sexual awareness and understanding, including the possibility of having conversations about sex.

Discussions about sexuality hold significant relevance in the upbringing of your child, and as a responsible parent, it is imperative for you to acknowledge this as a fundamental aspect of your responsibilities.

When you are engaged in retail therapy

Do you ever feel frustrated by the fact that gentlemen exhibit reluctance when it comes to accompanying us on shopping excursions? After engaging in a flirtatious exchange through text messages while shopping, he will eagerly express a desire to accompany you on future outings.

Visit a Victoria's Secret store and select some lingerie or athletic attire specifically designed for hot yoga practitioners (which tends to have a mesmerizing effect on many men). Please take a photograph of yourself while wearing an attractive pair of undergarments, such as a bikini, lingerie, or a one-piece swimsuit. This will demonstrate to him the reasons why he should accompany you on future shopping trips.

Some suggestive messages to exchange with him may comprise of:

May I ask for your advice on which attire I should acquire? Please provide him with a selection of images in advance.

Do you not desire to be present at this very moment, observing as I undergo a metamorphosis?

I long for your presence so that you may assist me in removing my garments...

What other options should I consider trying on?

Guidelines for capturing captivating images and videos to ignite his desire.

As previously stated, sexting entails more than the mere act of transmitting explicit messages.

In contemporary times, our cellular devices possess the ability to perform remarkable tasks. They possess the ability to capture photographs, record videos, and transmit vast amounts of data. Were you aware that contemporary smartphones possess a greater magnitude of computational capabilities as compared to the computers utilized for sending astronauts into space during the 1970s? That\\\'s crazy!

It would be highly illogical to overlook the opportunity to leverage the multitude of sophisticated functions available on your smartphone.

Enhance your sexting collection by including some provocative images and videos, resulting in an unparalleled level of sensual pleasure.

I have previously mentioned this, however, I feel compelled to reiterate: Exercise utmost caution in selecting individuals to whom you share images and videos. Engage in such behavior exclusively when you are in a committed relationship with a gentleman (or are legally wedded to him).

Okay, now, could you kindly enlighten me on the appropriate steps to capture alluring photographs and create sensual videos for the purpose of pleasing your significant other? Please continue reading below to discover the information.

Dildos

For reasons unknown, males exhibit heightened enthusiasm upon witnessing our engagement with personal pleasure devices, at least in my experience. Utilizing an intimate aid can be an exceptionally effective method to tantalize your partner. It will evoke strong sexual desire in him. He will be extremely eager to please you.

"Allow me to present several suggestions aimed at fostering his receptivity:

Capture an image of the phallic object tightly positioned next to your undergarments. Please transmit the image to him accompanied by a statement such as, "I yearn to possess your phallus in my grasp instead."

Place the phallic object within your vaginal area, while keeping your undergarments intact (albeit pulled aside). Please forward the following message to him: "I am becoming increasingly aroused in your presence."

Please capture an image depicting the act of placing your lips around the dildo. Please transmit the following message to him subsequently: "I desire to have the immediate pleasure of engaging in intimate activity with you."

Here are several explicit video illustrations:

Engage in oral stimulation with the phallic device to communicate your desire for his penis. Please express phrases similar to "I have a strong desire to experience your taste" or "I am interested in indulging in deep intimacy with you." Ensure that the video has a concise duration of three to four seconds.

*Please consider sharing with your spouse an intimate video of yourself engaging in self-pleasure. Please ensure to vocalize his name. Inform him of the extent to which you long for his presence.

Provocative images of intimate toys have the capacity to elicit highly sensual imaginings within his mind. Employ it solely when you have a strong desire for his presence.

Bananas (along with other edible items)

There seems to be a peculiar preoccupation among individuals of the male gender with foods that bear a resemblance to male genitalia, such as bananas and hotdogs."

Recently, during my time at the workplace, I inadvertently caught wind of a group of male individuals viewing a video depicting an attractive woman engaging in an action deemed provocative, in which she consumed a hotdog. I had to exert self-control in order to suppress my laughter.

Please capture an image while consuming the banana or hotdog. You will appear exceedingly pure, yet he will entertain unsettling notions.

Subsequently, communicate an explicit message to him via text. Please transmit a message of similar nature to him, such as:

I am currently consuming this banana. Would you like to engage in any activities later? :)

I express my desire for this to be under your ownership.

I have a strong appetite for poultry (albeit this might seem foolish, but it will highly excite him).

If you happen to possess the availability or possess the audacity, kindly record a video of yourself consuming the banana. Please ensure to fully insert it into your throat. Consume it gradually while expressing satisfaction through subtle sounds. That will immediately elicit a strong reaction from him.

Lips

For numerous gentlemen, a lady's lips possess an alluring and captivating quality. Consider the extent to which numerous individuals envision themselves with lips resembling those of Angelina Jolie.

Capture a few enticing images of your lips and forward them to him.

Allow me to present several suggestions:

Apply a sophisticated shade of lipstick, either in a striking red or a rich dark hue, and capture a close-up photograph. Kindly send him a subsequent text message conveying: "I eagerly anticipate our intimate encounter."

Apply gentle pressure to your lips using your teeth. Please send him a subsequent message stating: "You consistently elicit an arousal that leads to my involuntary lip-biting when we engage in intimacy."

Please capture an image in which you are gently touching your lips with your tongue. Kindly transmit the following message to him: "I am eagerly anticipating the moment to savor your presence."

Presented below are several trending video concepts:

Please capture a brief video wherein you delicately rotate your tongue over your lips, potentially accompanied by a subtle expression of pleasure. The video ought to have a duration of no more than three or four seconds. It\\\'ll drive him bananas.

Produce a video wherein you express your strong desire for him, ensuring to visually emphasize by zooming in on your attractive lips. Presented below, are a selection of statements:
I have an intense desire for your company.
-I miss your cock.
-I\\\'m waiting for you...

Crotch

Capturing an image of one's pelvic region serves as an exceptionally provocative gesture towards a male individual. Typically, I refrain from sharing photographs of my feline companion. I derive pleasure from playfully enticing my partner through selective exposure of either my undergarments or pants.

"Allow me to present several approaches to accomplish this task:

Capture an image of your denim attire and instruct him to conjecture the extent of moisture you have acquired. Once a response is received, remove your jeans and discreetly capture an image of your damp undergarments. This will prompt him to hurry home for intimacy with you!

"Capture an image of your fingers stimulating the clitoral region."

Communicate to him the challenges involved in patiently awaiting his return.

*Pull your panties all the way down to your ankles (take the photo from above looking down). I performed that act once for my significant other, eliciting a strong sensual response from him.

To effectively stimulate his disposition, consider reproducing the following video: "

Please recline on the bed and gently extend your legs apart. Caress your feline companion through the fabric of your undergarments and emit sounds of pleasure, potentially including the vocalization of the individual's name. Subsequently, deliver it to him...and additionally, contact the emergency medical services as a precautionary measure, as he may experience a loss of consciousness.

Legs

Numerous gentlemen appreciate the allure of a shapely set of legs on their female companion. Please take some photographs of your elegantly elongated legs for him, ensuring that you have carefully groomed them for obvious purposes :)

Below, I have provided a selection of alluring photographs that I have shared with my partner, causing him to experience intense fascination and desire.

Please adopt a seated posture where you place one leg over the other, either on a bench or on the table. Ensure sufficient illumination is provided so that he may adequately perceive the level of luster exhibited by them. He will be hurrying home to engage in intimate relations with you. Please transmit the following message to him subsequently to sending the image: 'I adore the manner in which you gently stroke your hands along my lower extremities...'

Would you mind capturing an image of yourself engaged in the act of shaving within the confines of the bathtub? Men are aware that women shave for a singular purpose.

For the purpose of creating an alluring video, assume a reclining posture on the bed, ensuring that your legs are parallel and neatly aligned. Next, massage your hands gently along your lower legs while playfully quipping, "Wouldn't you desire to experience the sensation of touching my velvety smooth legs?" Such an action is likely to evoke irresistible intrigue and fascination within him.

Inappropriate Discourse With Reserved Individuals

A considerable number of gentlemen exhibit significant reticence when it comes to engaging in explicit discourse. It is conceivable that they originate from a familial background characterized by conservative values, leading them to maintain a guarded attitude towards their sexual orientation. It is conceivable that other individuals may be waiting for your guidance due to their reluctance to appear unskilled in intimate situations. Furthermore, there are occasions when individuals of the male gender exhibit silence both in and outside the confines of intimate settings.

Prior to your arrival, it is possible that they had a previous romantic partner who desired a reticent demeanor during intimate moments. In the event that you encounter a reserved individual, it is imperative to attentively consider the underlying causes for their reticence in the bedroom, irrespective of the rationale. There is reason to be optimistic, whether it stems from a prior interpersonal connection or a deficit in experience. You have the ability to provide him with assistance and guidance throughout his journey. It is possible that he may gradually develop a greater level of ease in discussing explicit matters. Should his shyness stem from either his religious beliefs or a negative experience pertaining to his sexual development during his early years, it will pose considerable difficulty for him to alter his viewpoint. Commence at a gentle pace if you believe you have the capability to help your male partner overcome his reticence to engage in explicit communication. On the ensuing evening, during your next shared moment in bed, endeavor to communicate in a gentle manner to gauge his reaction. He is unlikely to reciprocate, so it is advisable to refrain from becoming discouraged. You may proceed as long as he manifests signs of enjoyment. It would be prudent to exercise caution and withdraw if he displays signs of physical unease or experiences a decline in his level of arousal. It is imperative to observe his response. If excessive pressure and hastiness are exerted, it is plausible that one could prevent him from engaging in vulgar speech indefinitely.

In addition to the confines of the bedroom, you may engage in conversation with your partner. Discover how he responds to explicit conversations and ascertain his personal preference towards such discussions. Inquire if his aversion to dirty talk stems from a genuine dislike or merely a fear of inadequate performance. Does he have any unarticulated thoughts due to his apprehension?

You are in a favorable position if your partner is receptive to the notion of engaging in intimate communication, yet experiences feelings of self-doubt concerning it. For both parties involved, aiding in his acquisition of provocative language can prove to be an enjoyable and mentally invigorating endeavor. You can effectively demonstrate your sentiments on the matter and offer constructive suggestions to enhance his self-assurance. The level of excitement during sexual experiences is expected to increase as his confidence grows, primarily through the incorporation of explicit verbal communication.

If you happen to discover that your male partner harbors strong personal or religious objections towards engaging in explicit conversations, it may be necessary to refrain from the use of explicit language. One can engage in conversations regarding his viewpoints and beliefs, but caution should be exercised to avoid unintentionally conveying an intention to alter his beliefs. Such a perception may lead to offense and discourage further participation in such discussions. Engage in a dialogue with him, subsequently determining the extent of your involvement. The potential benefit may not outweigh the associated risks. If you desire to maintain a positive relationship with the gentleman in question, it would be advisable to refrain from engaging in discussions of explicit or inappropriate nature.

Regarding the matter of engaging in explicit conversation, the majority of gentlemen simply require a slight nudge. They greatly appreciate it upon commencing. Initiate the conversation gradually and encourage your partner to discuss explicit subjects. It is imperative to consistently demonstrate deference towards his beliefs and attentively observe his conduct. Engaging in explicit conversation may not be favored by certain individuals. Do not attempt to coerce explicit conversation from your male counterpart if he demonstrates a reserved disposition towards such matters. It may be necessary for you to temporarily relinquish this desire, should you hold his value as a partner in high regard. If the usage of explicit language is significant to you, he might not possess qualities that align with your preferences.

Dirty Conversations

During Sex

Both genders partake in explicit conversations during sexual encounters, but how can one circumvent such interactions? It is conceivable that you have acquired considerable proficiency in engaging in sexting and amassing a fan base, yet the prospect of transposing those abilities into verbal communication is daunting. It is imperative to take into account factors such as the modulation of your voice, the selection of appropriate nicknames and phrases, among other considerations.

As previously mentioned, engaging in explicit conversations pertaining to sexual topics is deemed as inappropriate dialogue. However, there exist three distinct strategies that can be employed to cultivate a passionate atmosphere, namely: verbalizing one's emotions, assuming a dominant role, and diverting attention to arousing material that brings personal satisfaction. Narrating one's immediate sensations is considered one of the simplest approaches to indulge in explicit discourse. Do you encounter a sensation of cool tingling or pulsation? Inform your companion. When one communicates the current situation to their partner, it enhances the overall experience for both individuals and ensures that the information is conveyed concerning positive progress.

Sustain the dialogue for an extended period when nearing the point of reaching climax. It elicits excitement in your partner while intensifying the level of passion. One can choose to be either broad or detailed, depending on their progress in their exploration of provocative speech.

"I am unable to cease the act of kissing you," I uttered.

Presently, I am experiencing a sensation akin to jelly in my legs.

I am constantly preoccupied with thoughts of you.

She expressed a profound sense of proximity.

I expressed, "The movements of your tongue are driving me to a state of great fascination."

Your manual dexterity is exceptional.

You evoke a profound sense of significance within me.

I greatly cherish my profound connection with you.

\\\"I\\\'m so near. I find it repulsive. "I am on the verge of reaching climax."

Taking charge

Assuming a formal tone, an alternative way to express the same idea could be: "Exercising authority is both alluring and efficient." This represents an exemplary approach to engaging in erotic communication, as it is commonly observed that individuals of both genders often derive pleasure from experiencing dominance and receiving explicit guidance. Employ clear and straightforward communication. If your partner expresses a clear desire for increased physical assertiveness, then proceed accordingly. However, if their explicit preference in this regard is unclear or uncertain to you, simply assert yourself verbally. The following concepts are outlined below:

Currently, I desire your presence.

Bestow upon me a passionate embrace, surrendering your heart completely.

"He expressed a desire for your oral attention," he stated.

He expressed the desire for your oral attentiveness.

\\\"Rip my hair.\\\"

Engage in posterior intercourse with me upon inverting my position.

Please immobilize my arms by pinning them above my head.

I aspire to achieve professional excellence.

\\\"Scalp me.\\\"

Please transport me swiftly and efficiently.

Whether you choose to direct your attention towards me or not, is entirely your discretion.

\\\"Speak my name,\\\"

\\\"Cum for me.\\\"

Redirecting

Employing offensive language to guide your partner exhibits a semblance of assuming control. However, this observation is applicable solely when they are engaged in actions that do not genuinely resonate with you or when they struggle in executing a particular technique proficiently. This phenomenon is frequently observed in the context of oral intercourse, posing a difficulty for numerous individuals, especially those with limited prior experience. Your alluring voice provides them an alternative course of action instead of merely admonishing them with the phrase "Don't do that," which lacks motivation. It is imperative to remember to acknowledge and commend their actions when they exhibit appropriate behavior.

"Slower."

"Harder."

"Faster."

"Gently."

"Deeper."

\\\"Hold me closer.\\\"

May I inquire if you possess the ability to communicate orally?

"Higher."

"Lower."

I am fully ready for your presence.

\\\"Exactly like that.\\\"

"More."

\\\"Don\\\'t quit.\\\"

What if engaging in explicit language or sexual dialogue is not effectively enhancing the intimacy of the conversation?

When one is first embarking on the practice, engaging in explicit conversation can be uncomfortable. What if during intimate moments, the exploration of novel vocabulary and expressions proves ineffective? One possibility is that you are experiencing discomfort, or alternatively, your partner is not providing a response. Do not worry excessively! Keeping in mind that it is unnecessary to possess an extensive vocabulary of offensive remarks and that it is not obligatory to engage in constant conversation can significantly facilitate matters. The importance of quality prevails over quantity in this particular case. Should you find that using a limited amount of vulgar language during intimate occasions brings you the greatest comfort, please be assured that such behavior neither defines nor diminishes your worth. It would be inconvenient and disagreeable to enforce further imposition.

Do you happen to have any apprehensions about reiterating the same ideas repetitively? Expressions such as "This is truly remarkable," "I derive immense pleasure from the connection we share," or "My current attraction to you is insatiable" may not hold significance for your significant other. Your sincerity and passion will be discernible in your voice when you confidently express your genuine sentiments to your partner.

Furthermore, it is important to note that the response of your partner to dirty talk may not necessarily reflect their disinterest in it. They could potentially feel embarrassed and uncertain as to how to formulate a suitable reply. Inquire about their emotional state following the intimate encounter and emphasize the significance of receiving a spoken communication from them. Direct your attention to the auditory experiences if you happen to be the individual who is not highly vocal, yet still desires to communicate your enjoyment to your partner. Expressing audible pleasure is always encouraged, however, if you are aware that your partner desires explicit and provocative language, it may be advisable to incorporate some profanity into your discourse. These consist of assertive and concise expressions such as "Oh, expletive," "Expletive, indeed," and similar phrases. Phrases such as "Oh, God" are expected to be met with enthusiasm as well.

Video chat platforms like Skype provide individuals with the opportunity to engage in romantic encounters, facilitated by the advancements in technology. Such sexual experiences can be particularly advantageous for couples who are geographically separated or wherein one partner frequently embarks on travels, as they help maintain alignment in both their sexual and emotional connections. The trust between a couple is further solidified as they triumph over their initial discomfort and vulnerability. Proper Etiquette for Appropriate Language on Skype

Preparation

The vast majority of intimate activities via Skype do not transpire organically. This provides you with a sufficient amount of time to prepare and strategize the course of the session. This may involve making choices regarding your preferred intimate attire, a personal item or lubricant (should you desire to indulge yourself), curating a playlist, or creating an ambiance by lighting a candle. Moreover, it is crucial to strategize your course of action during this period. Are you planning to focus on recounting hypothetical scenarios of your interactions with your partner or on detailing your personal experiences and activities? May I inquire whether your significant other possesses a preferred term of endearment? A remark? Allocating one's efforts will enhance the intensity and enjoyment of virtual intimate encounters conducted over Skype.

Ensure that you can enjoy an uninterrupted setting, particularly if you have dependents or cohabitants, and approach it with the same reverence as a genuine romantic rendezvous. Are you capable of comprehending the extent of awkwardness that would ensue? Ideally, you will be afforded some uninterrupted hours of solitude within the comfort of your own dwelling. You are satisfied due to the fact that the door and windows have been closed. Henceforth, regard the Skype appointment with the same level of importance as a physical rendezvous. Please present yourself as if you were preparing for a sophisticated and alluring event in person. Please set aside your phone, switch off the television, and close any additional browser tabs in order to focus your undivided attention on your partner. Imagine that your associate is the sole remaining individual on the planet currently. Your vocal contribution holds immense significance. Please provide a description of your current activities and the activities that you desire to engage in. It is the epitome of closeness, as your partner is unable to physically make contact with you. In addition, their observation of your actions provides assistance, albeit it is the provocative quality of your tone that stimulates circulation. What particular declarations would you offer?

At present, you appear highly attractive, and my mind is filled with numerous plans involving you.

Are you ready for me to transition into wearing my undergarments?

I am currently completely soaked.

The current situation is extremely challenging.

I am firm in my handling of your hair while planting kisses on the nape of your neck.

She expressed that she could sense the motion of your hand caressing her, both upwards and downwards.

She expressed her imagination of being caressed by you orally.

I desire being enveloped by your essence/I long to experience the sensation of your presence within me.

Currently, my thoughts revolve around envisioning you engaging in intense and passionate activity with me.

In formal tone one could say, "Inappropriate discussions conducted via Skype are often complemented by a variety of auditory elements, such as audible discomfort and heavy breathing." They will promptly induce a state of sensuality in your mind. If you are uncertain about what to express, you could consider engaging in the recitation of literary works with romantic or sensual themes. If one derives pleasure from writing, they may consider developing their erotic conversation in advance and deliver it verbally to ensure its authenticity and to establish with their partner that it stems from their own thoughts.

Following sexual activity, there is no requirement for inappropriate conversation to cease. This approach serves as an effective means to foster a sense of intimacy, facilitate communication, and provide constructive input on one's preferences. Furthermore, now would be an opportune moment to discuss the activities you may wish to explore in future instances of passionate intimacy. Some examples include:

She stated that her knees remained feeble.

I am experiencing dizziness and disorientation.

"I am uncertain whether I am capable of remaining upright for an extended period," I voice.

I greatly admired the auditory expressions you were generating.

\\\"When you... (expressed or performed this specific action), it exuded a strong sense of allure.

She expressed her delight in the fact that she could still perceive your flavor.

She expressed the need to address that matter during our upcoming encounter.

Tomorrow, "I shall ponder upon that incessantly."

I desire that our current state endures indefinitely.

Actions to Avoid

We have provided you with several illustrative methods of engaging in explicit communication, however, are there any prohibitions or restrictions to be mindful of when endeavoring to employ these techniques with your partner? Here are the three primary principles:

Refrain from eliciting laughter from your partner.

Engaging in inappropriate dialogue can create discomfort, particularly when it is unfamiliar. Your counterpart might still be in the process of acclimating to your manner of speaking and choice of words, while you may already be quite comfortable with them. You may experience bouts of laughter when they generate comical or lighthearted content. Resist. Your partner will remain silent as a result of their fear of appearing foolish, as laughter would elicit that feeling. They may lack any inclination to engage in the arduous conversation once more. In order to explore alternative possibilities, instead of amusement, kindly propose alternative statements or share a preferred name.

It is advisable to refrain from uttering any profanities or engaging in explicit discussions when exposed to explicit content, as well as to avoid experimenting with such language.

You may encounter words or phrases that you find unsatisfactory. However, your partner may potentially provide a favorable response. Despite your aversion to referring to your partner as a derogatory term, it appears that they derive pleasure from it and are desirous of you intensifying your assertiveness. It might be alluring to circumvent the discussion of your discomfort due to your partner's satisfaction. This situation could potentially have a significant detrimental impact on your relationship. You may experience a sense of deception, or even more distressing emotions. Your ability to genuinely enjoy the intimate experience with your partner may be hindered due to considerable discomfort, thus having adverse effects on the both of you. Speak with them. An agreement can be reached.

Exercise caution and refrain from hastening.

Provocative discourse, encompassing a multitude of nuances and complexities. Despite individuals potentially having a sense of the level of extremity they desire, a significant portion of the population tends to opt for a gradual approach. This proposition is commendable as it facilitates a mutually beneficial opportunity for you and your partner to acquire a comprehensive understanding of each other's individual aptitudes and limitations. Engaging in hasty actions can be overwhelming and result in unsettling, if not disturbing, situations that cast a detrimental perception upon the use of vulgar language. If you and your partner have recently initiated your romantic relationship, exercising prudence and vigilance assumes particular significance. You are still in the process of building trust among individuals. Simply remain calm and patient.

How to Cultivate Influence and Assertiveness in Interactions with Women

There is nothing more intimidating for a gentleman who harbors feelings for a young lady than to be met with her refusal. It is something worth contemplating. This minuscule lexeme has rendered innumerable individuals into anxious wrecks. No one would refute the arduous nature of experiencing rejection, however, it is imperative to maintain a perspective. If one truly desires to achieve success yet continues to struggle, it may be opportune to alter one's approach before all the desirable opportunities dissipate.

PITFALLS TO BE AVOIDED WHEN INTERACTING WITH WOMEN

Error #1: Failing to Depart the Residences (Or Dwelling)

Initiate contact with women at once. Women are not inclined to approach you. The most effective approach to initiating the process of acquiring confidence in interacting with women is to actively engage in public situations and conscientiously refine one's social aptitude. Engage in conversation with individuals of all genders, and endeavor to be socially outgoing. With increasing frequency of performing this activity, it will gradually become less challenging. In due course, you will inevitably encounter situations that you currently perceive as lacking. Frequently engaging in activities also invariably enhances the likelihood of favorable outcomes occurring in your life. There is a surplus of individuals in society, including myself in the past, who would enhance their self-assurance with women more expeditiously through increased social engagement. I understand that this may appear to be self-evident, but believe me, a significant transformation occurred in my life when I came to the realization that I no longer required further engagement in reading, studying, attending seminars, or consuming educational materials.

Do not be the individual who feels compelled to possess comprehensive knowledge on seduction techniques before taking action in meeting attractive women. You will never acquire comprehensive knowledge prior to commencing. Engaging in the practical application of acquired knowledge concurrently enhances the learning process and fosters a more comprehensive understanding.

Error #2: Excessive Concern Regarding a Woman's Thoughts and Perceptions Towards Them.

Dear individuals, it is indeed a colossal blunder to become entangled in the confines of one's own thoughts. These factors will undermine your success in numerous ways. Here is a rather ironic revelation that I came across a couple of years ago: I receive a greater number of unfavorable responses from women when, within my thoughts, I deliberate extensively on what I should articulate prior to expressing it. This matter holds significant importance, thus I kindly request you to contemplate this for a moment. When I engage in the rapid cognitive process (typically lasting 2-3 seconds) of internal contemplation and strategizing an optimal verbal response, it often elicits unfavorable reactions, not only from females but males as well. Why is this? The reason for their perception is that they are able to discern that your approach is based on a sense of dependency, thus emphasizing the significance of ensuring that your words are received positively. What is paradoxical, of course, is that the desire for something to succeed often leads to its inevitable failure.

In a sociocultural setting, individuals typically aim to avoid experiencing discomfort or being in the presence of someone who exhibits signs of dependency, even if such indications are nuanced as demonstrated in this particular instance. It makes people uncomfortable. However, this location serves as a significantly superior destination for one to arrive from:

I am confident that the majority of the time, I have valuable insights to contribute. Therefore, I will respond spontaneously and instinctively, without excessive deliberation. If my responses are not well-received, I accept that outcome, as I am aware that they are usually appreciated.

This frame elicits a subconscious response that induces a sense of increased relaxation among individuals in your presence. You aren\\\'t "needing" anything. Consider this scenario: while dining with someone, if their meal takes an excessively long time to be served, your discomfort intensifies in direct proportion to their persistent demands regarding their order. The situation remains unchanged when a woman engages in conversation with a man who has a subconscious desire for his words to be amusing; it simply occurs to a lesser extent. Do not concern yourself with the opinions of others. If you possess exemplary qualities, it is highly probable that a woman of similar caliber will acknowledge and appreciate your worth.

Error #3: Transforming Rejection into Reality

Allow me to impart a confidential insight I have acquired regarding cultivating self-assurance when engaging with women: The notion of rejection is merely a construct of one's own imagination. A belief is a cognitive construct that is actualized by an individual. As you have matured, society has instilled within you the notion that encountering rejection is an inherent possibility, manifesting itself in various ways. You have taken this idea and given it substance by transforming it into a conviction.

You developed an unquestioning belief in your early years that being rejected is possible and must be diligently avoided. The aforementioned cycle occurred when you conceived the notion that you possess 'a lack of trust in women.' This was solidified through the transformation of that thought into a belief.

Denial lacks substantive validity, for upon contemplation, one must consider the absence of any tangible loss. You did not possess her interest prior to initiating contact, and you currently do not possess it. You have not incurred any losses. However, Ash, the issue at hand pertains not to safeguarding what I currently possess, but rather to acquiring something that I do not yet possess. In response to that, I assert that the intense yearning for her validation arises once more. Why, I am compelled to inquire, do you find such a desperate need for her approval? Why can't you simply engage in social interactions and make an effort to present yourself, and if she shows interest, then that would be excellent and fortunate. When originating from a state of insignificance, it becomes infeasible to experience rejection. Allow me to reiterate:

When one originates from a state of self-sufficiency, the prospect of facing rejection becomes implausible.

Mistake #4: Erroneously Assuming That Confidence Is an Innate Trait Possessed by All Men Who Achieve Success in Their Interactions with Women

Although it is accurate that individuals possess unique personalities and some individuals are fortunate to naturally exude self-confidence with women, it should be noted that this does not imply one cannot cultivate these traits within themselves. Acquiring confidence when interacting with females is an acquirable aptitude that can be developed, resulting in personal growth. Consider, for example, the proficiency in playing a musical instrument, such as the guitar. Every individual who possesses exceptional guitar skills underwent a learning process in order to acquire proficiency in playing the instrument.

Developing self-confidence is an acquirable and refineable skillset that can be cultivated with the passage of time. My utmost recommendation would be to actively engage in conversations with individuals on a frequent basis. The more expeditiously you acquire the skill of socializing with individuals, the swifter you shall develop self-assurance in your interpersonal relationships. This assertion holds particular significance when it comes to women. Additional strategies that can be employed to enhance one's rapport with women encompass: Engaging in physical fitness regimens to achieve optimal physical condition, vocalizing affirmations regularly to oneself, and employing visual exercises utilizing NLP techniques (Neuro-Linguistic Programming).

Mistake #5: Failing to Harness the Influence of Non-Verbal Communication and Body Language

Oftentimes, it is the simplest factors that yield the most significant impact. Research has evidenced that a substantial majority, ranging between 80% to 90%, of our interpersonal communication relies on non-verbal cues. To put it differently, non-verbal communication. It would greatly behoove you to dedicate time to the study of body language. One can effectively convey multiple messages simultaneously through nonverbal cues, making body language an immensely influential means of communication. Are you of the opinion that one can glean substantial insights about an individual based on their choice of attire? Naturally, the information you compile is subject to change, but for the most part, it is typically quite precise. Body language functions in a similar manner. Below, you will find a collection of invaluable suggestions pertaining to the mastery of body language:

- Initiating and maintaining visual contact

- Engaging in more deliberate motions - Adopting a more measured pace - Executing actions with greater restraint

- Conducting movements at a reduced speed - Implementing a more restrained approach to physical actions

- Demonstrating a lower level of reactivity towards others compared to their level of reactivity towards you

- Maintaining an upright posture with shoulders slightly retracted

- Expressing a pleasant facial gesture

- Remaining upright or keeping one's distance while engaging in conversation with her.

- Modulating voice pitch and pace (e.g., avoiding rapid speech and incorporating pauses). This is unrelated to the verbal expression or the communicated message.

Error #6: Obtaining her contact details without a clear objective

There was once a period in my past where I, like many inexperienced individuals, held the belief that obtaining a person's phone number guaranteed their complete attention and interest. This assertion is entirely far removed from reality. Having a phone number serves no practical purpose unless there is a specific motive for obtaining it. One common error that I have noticed is when individuals inquire about the phone number prematurely. In reality, she is so accustomed to men engaging in this behavior that she is likely desensitized to it. Thus, when you approach her, she has become socially conditioned to simply provide her number, similar to how she did with the preceding ten individuals.

To be candid, it would typically require a considerable lack of skill or charm not to obtain her contact information within a five-minute conversation. Unmarried, aesthetically pleasing women frequently disclose their contact information; the distinction lies in the manner in which you request it.

Consider the following perspective: "I will approach this situation by giving this woman an opportunity to become acquainted with me. If I determine that she would be enjoyable to spend time with, I will arrange a meeting and obtain her contact information during that process." Unless pressed for time, it is strongly recommended to engage in a conversation with her for a duration of at least 7-12 minutes, in order to establish a modest familiarity with her, before scheduling a meeting and acquiring her contact details. Consider it as if she has successfully met your criteria of being "cool," and her reward is that you intend to request her contact information (while making arrangements). Embracing this perspective will also facilitate the development of your confidence when interacting with women in general, as you gain experience and refine your skills.

Error #7: Failing to Approach or Initiate when the Opportunity Presents Itself.

Have you managed to depart from your residence? Excellent! However, it is imperative that you acquire the knowledge of effectively encountering captivating women in social settings. Engaging in social activities while passively holding a beer against your chest will not yield any positive outcomes. Females will not initiate an approach towards you. In upscale occasions, it is not uncommon for attractive gentlemen who are elegantly attired to be approached by women. Nevertheless, it remains the responsibility of the man to seize the opportunity and engage in conversation with them. You must cease your incessant preoccupation with potential negative outcomes by examining and exposing her. Acknowledge and embrace the fact that there is a strong possibility that you may encounter her in a negative frame of mind or during an inconvenient moment, and that is perfectly acceptable.

In most instances, if one were to approach with a pleasant facial expression, positive non-verbal cues, and confident vocal modulation, it is highly probable that she would be receptive to engaging in conversation. Women anticipate being approached when they go out, particularly those who are visually appealing. They have grown accustomed to men seeking their company, so it is not a significant matter. In alternative terms, it is not as if you are engaging in anything unconventional or unconventional by approaching her. Please make an effort to adapt yourself to the given circumstance, and be aware that approaching her from behind is not advisable. However, what holds significance is that you possess the mindset: Approach Women Now.

Flaw #8: Insufficient employment of humor (or complete absence thereof) during interactions with her.

I cannot overemphasize the significance of incorporating humor as a crucial element in the process of building confidence and rapport with women. Please refrain from interpreting this as an invitation to engage in excessive rumination or hastily formulate humorous remarks or clever one-liners.

What I am trying to convey here is adopting a relaxed and effortless demeanor, and seizing the occasions to exhibit cleverness as they arise. A young woman typically presents numerous occasions to engage in light-hearted banter and playfully tease her during an interaction. After practicing this technique multiple times, you will inherently enhance your ability and acquire the proficiency to identify these opportunities.

Women are fond of men who possess the ability to engage in light-hearted teasing and banter, demonstrating an absence of fear in doing so, while simultaneously exhibiting the capacity to graciously accept such jesting from their female counterparts. It indicates your high level of social intelligence and your ability to understand social dynamics. It demonstrates your self-assurance in interactions with women. It also enhances the enjoyment and creates a more relaxed atmosphere during the interaction. Also remember that much like conversation, humor is not linear, meaning if you tease her about something, you can loop back to it again at a later point and tease her again about it. This fosters a perception of mutual rapport and profound comprehension between the two of you, an aspect of substantial magnitude.

Individuals who are not acquainted with one another to a significant extent are improbable to establish a connection of a similar nature and engage in communication on such a profound level. It is intriguing to note that even with a mere acquaintance of 5 minutes, if one has the ability to engage with her on this level (employing socially intelligent humor, playfully teasing her, etc.), she will perceive a sense of familiarity as if the bond has been established over a significantly longer period of time.

Error #9: Granting women control over their emotional responses via the remote control.

An attribute associated with femininity, as observed in the female persona, is its inherent variability, akin to the dynamic nature of weather patterns. Females are inclined to experience a broader range of moods and emotional fluctuations compared to males. One common error observed among individuals of the male gender is that when faced with a slightly challenging situation or a remark intended to provoke, men often permit such occurrences to adversely impact their mood or current emotional disposition. This is a matter that personally required a significant amount of time for me to comprehend and appropriately address.

This is also among the more sophisticated and arduous skills that you will acquire in the process of developing confidence with women.

Although it is a slightly more advanced skill, it remains of utmost importance to promptly comprehend and address it. Do not allow a comment, opinion, or minor fluctuation in mood to alter your positive emotional state or disposition. A lady must be aware, particularly when evaluating you as a potential romantic partner, that you possess the capability to adeptly handle challenging situations when she becomes somewhat disagreeable. It is incumbent upon you, as an aligned, resolute individual, to possess the capacity to manage these situations without exhibiting excessive reactions or allowing them to have an impact on you. If you respond with excessive emotional reactions or agitation during these occurrences, you are essentially behaving in an immature manner. Please keep in mind that when she is behaving childishly, it is necessary for you to maintain your strength and exhibit maturity, rather than allowing yourself to regress into an immature state. If you happen to do so, then both individuals involved will find themselves in an unfavorable situation. It is imperative to bear in mind that a woman requires the companionship of a mature man, rather than an immature juvenile.

Error #10: Regarding and dealing with a woman as a trophy to be acquired rather than as an individual.

This is a concept that is so straightforward that it can be easily overlooked (or even fail to be acknowledged initially). It is crucial to consistently bear in mind, particularly when in the company of attractive individuals, that they are simply ordinary individuals. Beneath their appealing exterior, they exhibit no variation from any other individual. They experience apprehensions and uncertainties; they become anxious, emotional, and self-conscious, similar to how men occasionally do. Keeping this in mind will dismantle the pedestal upon which you have placed her in your mind solely due to her physical appearance (treating her as an object to be won).

It is quite effortless to be ensnared by the physical appearance of an appealing woman. Women do not commonly encounter this issue with men, at least not frequently. Ultimately, what a woman desires from you is to cease inundating her with excessive displays of affection, compliments, and attention, but instead to regard her as the individual she truly is: a human being. She will show greater receptivity to your affection, praise, and compliments if they originate from a basis of sincerity (after you have acquainted yourself with her to some extent) rather than if you convey them hastily and in a manner that is nearly identical to how the previous ten individuals did.

How to overcome shyness and cultivate a high level of confidence when interacting with women

Tip 1: Adopting a Relaxed Demeanor. Even if you do not perceive a distinct change in the situation, it is advisable to endeavor to present yourself in a composed manner.

Please be mindful of the fact that there are numerous other women available, and therefore, if you happen to miss an opportunity with one particular individual, there will be an abundance of other prospects to consider. However, in the event that you have a specific goal in mind, it would be advisable to project an image of mild disinterest regarding her. Women generally do not find men appealing when they display overly possessive and desperate behavior.

Tip 2: "Visualization." Picture yourself in a scenario where you find yourself amidst a group of females. Consider oneself to possess great courage and lacking any issues with self-assurance. Immerse yourself in this scenario and endeavor to adapt to real life.

Tip 3: "Transfer of Authority." Another effective approach to surmount self-confidence challenges is to refrain from granting the woman in question the authority to decline your advances. In conjunction with the initial suggestion, it will be observed that if one does not appear excessively enthusiastic but rather maintains just the right amount of engagement in conversation, one will find that the anticipation in the atmosphere will lead to her heightened excitement, potentially resulting in her pursuit of you if you execute the process correctly.

Can The Practice Of Hypnosis Enhance One's Self-Assurance And Ease In Interpersonal Interactions With Women?

Confidence is an intriguing aspect, and when it pertains to achieving success with women, it holds paramount significance. A contributing factor lies within our delineation of the true essence of confidence. One can effectively engage in dialogue and assume the role of a conversation leader. If you possessed the requisite knowledge and skills to consistently perform this task, it is likely that you would exhibit a significantly higher level of confidence. There is also the concept of self-esteem or self-worth. Men who are perceived as possessing a sense of "assurance" are commonly regarded as being considerably more appealing to women. This presents a significantly greater challenge to falsify. Any individual possesses the potential to acquire a sufficient repertoire of scripts, techniques, or performances to feign expertise, but if one genuinely lacks conviction in their worthiness of engaging with this lady, their endeavors are destined for failure.

This is where hypnosis can assist you. All individuals possess both appealing and unappealing aspects in their personal characteristics. Through the skillful application of self-hypnosis, one can cultivate an assortment of positive personality traits without necessitating any alteration of their fundamental identity. An exceptional method that I impart to individuals is characterized by its remarkable efficacy and simplicity. The sequence is as follows:

Initially, begin by documenting all the attributes and characteristics you desire in women. Please provide a comprehensive account of the sensations and experiences one would encounter upon possessing these qualities. You must envision with utmost clarity the sensations you will experience when engaging in confident conversations with women.

Amplify and enhance these emotions or visuals at present. Immerse yourself in the perspective of that individual and perceive the world through the lens of your ideal self.

It is advisable to perform this exercise on a daily basis, whether you are in a vehicle, on public transportation, or during any available leisure time. The greater amount of practice you engage in, the higher level of proficiency you will attain. The objective is to enhance the overall visualization process to its fullest potential.

The methodology is effective due to the inability of your subconscious mind to distinguish between actual and simulated occurrences. By engaging in this technique, one can manipulate their subconscious into perceiving synthetic encounters with women as genuine successes. The more vivid the visualization, the more authentic it will be perceived by the subconscious mind. Likewise, the subconscious mind is prone to fixate on the concept of being rejected, thus it is advisable to refrain from entertaining such thoughts.

Cease relying on self-assurance with women, acquire proficiency.
Let us examine the definitions once more:
Confidence: complete faith; conviction in the competence, credibility, or dependability of an individual or entity: We possess unwavering confidence in their capacity to achieve success.
Competence is defined as the state or quality of being competent, indicating adequacy and possession of the necessary skills, knowledge, qualifications, or capacity. The reason for hiring her was due to her competence in the field of accountancy.
The first proposition is based on the foundation of faith and reliance, whereas the second proposition is based on the substantiation and validation. The allure

of confidence is readily evident to men compared to women.

Attaining competency necessitates diligent effort and consistent practice. Acquiring knowledge, perusing literature, and observing visual resources can never serve as a substitute for practical experience. When we exhibit proficiency, we embody it in every aspect of our being and every action we undertake. Confidence serves only to make an impression, yet it lacks the substantial evidence required for validity.

To transition from confidence to competence necessitates taking proactive measures. One becomes proficient in driving through the act of driving. Engaging in driving without prior practice would be highly risky and potentially life-threatening. That is precisely the reason why we engage in examinations, why we diligently refine our golf swings, and why we persistently repeat our actions. By consistently repeating activities, we internalize them, seamlessly integrating them into our conduct until they become intrinsic and proficient.

Therefore, considering this fact, how can you implement it in your interactions with women? One can commence by acknowledging that each rejection brings us one step closer to acceptance. Find satisfaction in the knowledge that, reiterate it to yourself prior to engaging in any form of communication with females. Rejection serves as constructive feedback rather than a personal attack. Envision a scenario in which you have recently encountered an individual at a social establishment. The exchange did not transpire in the manner you had hoped, as she exhibited disrespectful behavior towards you. Can this be seen as an indication of your character? or hers? I apologize if my words come across as blunt, but it is important to understand that removing personal emotions from the situation is invaluable advice. Consider this: Do professional tennis players engage in negative self-talk and relinquish their efforts if they happen to lose a match?

No, it is evident that they have suffered significant losses, amounting to potentially hundreds or even thousands of matches.
Being a professional entails experiencing failure on numerous occasions.
Possessing a high level of proficiency in interacting with women implies that one has confronted numerous instances of refusal or dismissal. Arriving at a tennis court adorned in the latest fashion trends and equipped with modern gear might enhance your outward confidence, yet the true assessment of your skill lies within the performance of your game. Engage in outdoor activities and leverage constructive feedback to your advantage.

Understanding Emotional And Cultural Consent: Its Significance And Relevance

In the realm of tantric sexuality, as with any other manifestation of intimate physical connection, consent is a fundamental prerequisite. However, there exists a slight variation on this occasion.

The Essence of Consent: An Intriguing Perspective on its Allure

Consent is an essential factor that should be present in the interactions of the majority of individuals. It not only facilitates mutually advantageous engagement in sexual situations but also serves as a fundamental distinction between consensual intercourse and instances of sexual assault or mistreatment.

Securing consent is an imperative that necessitates continual effort. The majority of individuals lack comprehension regarding the profound consequences of engaging in nonconsensual activities, whether of a sexual nature or otherwise. The presence of consent, however, grants individuals the ability to willingly expose themselves to such activities, thereby enhancing their overall well-being and contentment.

However, consent extends beyond the realm of physicality. The complete acceptance of physical contact in that specific area carries significant weight, but it encompasses more than mere physical behavior.

Additionally, it can be described as a comprehensive and encompassing agreement that pertains to emotional, psychological, and sociocultural aspects.

In the majority of relationships, physical consent is typically granted. You express acceptance of engaging in sexual activity, and subsequently engage in it. However, tantric sex necessitates the presence of emotional and cultural consent, two crucial elements that are typically absent in conventional sexual experiences. Sexual intercourse can evoke deep emotional responses, however, typically, explicit emotional consent is not always necessary during such activities. However, in the realm of tantra, it is an endeavor that involves profound emotional engagement. It is imperative to comprehend that, in order to derive utmost fulfillment from the practice of tantra, one must willingly grant permission to explore and embrace both personal and interpersonal emotions.

What Does the Concept of Emotional Consent Entail?

Emotional consent pertains to granting approval for the emotions communicated by someone else, or those which you express yourself.

Have you ever engaged in a conversation where initially you are discussing a personal issue, but then your acquaintance unexpectedly interjects with uninvited guidance on how to navigate the situation? Have you previously engaged in this activity? Frequently, the significance of obtaining emotional consent is equivalent to that of physical consent. It is unfavorable to align oneself with either party involved in such interactions, as engaging in them frequently leads to unsatisfactory conversations and subsequent frustration for the majority of individuals.

The issue lies in the inherent complexity of our existence, and it is essential to comprehend the necessity of establishing profound interpersonal bonds with individuals whom we encounter. However, it is essential that you provide your consent to undergo such emotional experiences. Engaging in alternative actions enables the establishment of trust with the other individual, while also providing a platform for the exchange of thoughts and ideas.

Engaging in conversation with others can be exhausting. Engaging in emotional labor is not typically a voluntary commitment for many individuals, and thus, emotional consent gains paramount significance as it upholds the recognition of granting another person the opportunity to comprehend one's perspective. Consequently, it serves to prevent overwhelming others with an influx of emotions, enabling both parties to establish and maintain healthy and contented boundaries in their interactions with others.

Obtaining emotional consent is contingent upon mutual agreement to embrace and experience its repercussions, thereby yielding potential advantages for both parties involved.

Emotional consent extends beyond a mere inclination to lend an ear to someone's problems. Frequently in the practice of tantra, emotional consent involves giving oneself permission to be confronted with the more challenging aspects of the world.

When engaging in the practice of tantra, individuals undergo a plethora of emotions and frequently necessitate mutual alignment in their perspectives. Engaging in synchronized respiration, maintaining visual contact, and attuning to each other's energy can prove challenging, particularly following a prolonged period of activity. Hence, it is crucial, in the practice of tantric sex, to engage in it during a state of unburdened detachment from the distractions of daily life. This will allow for a heightened receptiveness and effective application of the knowledge attained about one's partner.

Engaging in this particular practice is highly imbued with spirituality, and one must willingly give permission to delve into such profound emotional states. On occasion, when engaging in this behavior as well, one encounters distressing issues.

Addressing Trauma and Ensuring Emotional Consent

The sentiments one undergoes during the practice of tantric sex transcend individual emotions, encompassing the shared emotional landscape of both partners. Tantric sexual practices aim to facilitate liberation from interpersonal constraints and are frequently accompanied by the realization that, contrary to general perception, engaging in tantric sex can be an immensely invigorating and mutually enhancing experience.

Tantalic sexual practices encompass the examination of psychological associations and traumas related to the act of sexual engagement as well. For a significant number of individuals, there is a tendency to neglect the opportunity to derive pleasure from the present moment, as well as the ensuing emotional experiences. However, by engaging in tantric practices, we can transcend the challenges of our previous experiences, thereby empowering us to confront the future. Nevertheless, it is imperative to comprehend that this phenomenon has the capacity to evoke strong emotions, presenting both positive prospects and considerable burdens. Appreciate that when engaging in tantric sex, you are inherently exposing yourself to the emotional distress and challenges experienced by your partner, a fact that often goes unnoticed leading to an incomplete grasp of the immense potential of tantric practices. For the majority of individuals, engaging in tantric sexual practices facilitates a deeper comprehension of one's own individual well-being and an enhanced capacity to earnestly delve into uncharted territories.

It is imperative to acknowledge the significance of granting one's consent, particularly in the context of tantric sexual activities. It is crucial to comprehend that consent must be voluntarily given, informed, accompanied by genuine enthusiasm, and established through effective communication with the participating individual.

Engaging in communication, particularly in the midst of distressing circumstances, could prove beneficial for your well-being. It enables individuals to explore their desires and emotions in a manner that promotes wellbeing. Please bear in mind that you are also considering the exploration and removal of sexual boundaries, allowing for personal liberation and the enhancement of your overall well-being and contentment. Obtaining consent is highly beneficial not only for examining the emotional dimensions of an individual, but also for addressing trauma associated with this matter, which is more prevalent than one might realize.

Incorporating Consent into Our Cultural Framework

Tantric sexual practices promote wholehearted consent to all actions undertaken. That is the prevailing cultural norm associated with it. When embarking upon the practice of tantra, the ultimate objective is liberation, necessitating one's acceptance of the premise that engaging in tantra entails encounters with novel experiences that may significantly impact individuals.

It is imperative for you to comprehend the importance of advocating for yourself and expressing your own individual sentiments. It is imperative to exercise critical thinking and independent judgment rather than unquestioningly adhering to doctrines. Moreover, in the event of practicing tantra under the guidance of an experienced individual, it is equally important to engage in personal reflection and draw one's own conclusions. It is advisable to adhere to your comfort zones when it comes to engaging with tantra, as this approach can help mitigate the likelihood of experiencing subsequent feelings of remorse.

It is imperative to consistently communicate your limits when engaging in tantric sexual practices. If you prefer the sensation of being touched in certain areas and not in others, it is advisable to always inform the individual accompanying you of your preferences.

It is imperative that you comprehend that engaging in collective coercion is also strictly prohibited. One should never feel obligated to undertake a task simply due to societal expectations or commands. Certain individuals excel in engaging in discussion, and in the context of tantra, it is encouraged to partake in open and honest dialogue with one's partner to foster mutual understanding and alignment.

When practicing tantra, it is imperative to establish a reliable system for honest feedback during the process. Should you have any dislikes, it is advisable to communicate them to your partner. Equally important is expressing any preferences or likes you may have. It is imperative to consistently prioritize mutual agreement and ensure harmonious alignment with your partner.

And, as customary, it is imperative to recognize that tantra is an inherently individualistic pursuit. There is no necessity to vociferously disclose the details of your extended five-hour tantric sexual encounter to others. It is imperative that the matter be confined to private discussion between the two of you, rather than being openly disclosed. Maintain the utmost discretion concerning this matter, as it will contribute to enhancing both the quality of the intimate experience and the overall well-being shared between individuals.

Boundaries Retain Relevance within the Realm of Tantra

Lastly, it is crucial to maintain clear boundaries in the context of tantric sexual practices. This is due to the fact that despite the dynamics of tantric sex emphasizing spontaneity and engaging both the mind and body, it is imperative to acknowledge and respect certain limitations that ought not to be surpassed.

If such a violation were to occur, it would be deemed unacceptable. That act constitutes assault, which is an occurrence that should never transpire. Alternatively, adopt a policy of sincerity towards your significant other, while also ensuring that boundaries are appropriately communicated and established to accommodate all parties involved, taking into consideration their well-being and security.

As is customary, akin to any other form of sexual encounter, it is crucial to uphold consent and strive for a consensual and collaborative approach. It is strongly recommended that you also take the initiative to acquire a thorough comprehension of the significance of consent, along with its implications when mutually expressed with your partner. Initiate a thorough discussion on this matter at an early stage while ensuring diligent resolution of both the logistical and emotional aspects, as well as the nature of the cultural authorization that will be obtained.

Cultural consent can manifest through various expressions, such as incorporating ritualistic practices or donning attire that symbolizes shared cultural value. It is imperative to engage in pre-discussions with your partner to establish mutual understanding and alignment, as this step alone can significantly enhance your overall experience.

Middle Childhood

Our bodies

Familiarize yourself with appropriate terminology when discussing anatomical structures of the human body, encompassing both male and female individuals. This includes employing the corresponding terms for genitalia such as the penis, testicles, scrotum, anus, vulva, labia, vagina, clitoris, uterus, and ovaries.

To possess a certain level of familiarity with the internal anatomical structures associated with reproduction, including the uterus, ovaries, fallopian tubes, urethra, bladder, and bowel.

Those bodies exhibit a diverse range of shapes, sizes, and colors. Both male and female individuals possess anatomical features that can elicit pleasurable sensations upon physical contact.

To possess the capacity to attend to one's own physical well-being, including the proper care of their bodily features such as intimate areas, hair, teeth, skin, and so forth.

To possess effective techniques for declining – "Cease your actions, as they are not to my liking."

Puberty

That their physiological makeup will undergo modifications as they advance in age.

Puberty entails both physiological and psychological transformations. If a comprehensive understanding of the alterations is desired, it is apropos to discuss the transcendence occurring during this phase, as individuals progress towards adulthood.

Sexual intercourse

The occurrence of conception arises from the union of a man's sperm with a woman's ovum, typically transpiring through sexual intercourse (in vitro fertilization represents an alternative method).

The process of conception occurs when seminal fluid is expelled from the male reproductive organ and subsequently enters the female reproductive organ. Subsequently, they navigate towards the location where the egg is situated. The process entails the fusion of the egg and sperm, subsequently leading to the development of a fetus.

It is a widely acknowledged fact that adults engage in sexual activities, which is considered a natural, ordinary, and beneficial aspect of human existence. Adults frequently engage in acts of physical affection such as kissing, embracing, and engaging in other intimate behaviors as means of expressing affection and seeking personal satisfaction. Sexual intercourse is an act intended for adults and is not appropriate for children.

The decision of whether or not to conceive rests with the individual of mature age.

Sexual behavior

Masturbation is a behavior that varies among children, with some engaging in it and others refraining from doing so. It is expected that all sexual conduct remains confidential, including acts such as masturbation and sexual intercourse. The sensation experienced when coming into contact with that physique can be highly pleasurable.

Occasionally, individuals may peruse explicit imagery or content depicting nudity and sexual activities on the internet, which is unsuitable for a young audience. In addition, it is imperative to engage in a conversation with your child regarding the appropriate actions they should take upon encountering such images, without presuming that they will inevitably come across them.

Elucidate the existence of diverse sexual orientations, encompassing individuals who identify as heterosexual, homosexual, or bisexual.

Love

Love signifies experiencing profound and affectionate sentiments towards oneself and individuals around. Individuals have the capacity to encounter various manifestations of affection. Individuals demonstrate affection in various manners towards their parents, familial relations, and acquaintances. Dating refers to a situation in which two individuals develop a romantic attraction towards one another and engage in activities during their leisure hours. Adolescence marks the commencement of romantic relationships.
Individuals can encounter diverse affectionate connections over the course of their lifetimes.

Friendships

One can possess numerous companions or only a small number.
One may acquire various types of friendships. Despite the occurrence of conflicts, friendships can endure even when individuals experience anger towards one another.
Companions engage in shared activities and develop familiarity with one another.

Acquaintances have the capacity to inflict emotional harm upon one another. Friendships depend on honesty. Companions can vary in age and gender, encompassing individuals who are both older and younger, as well as both male and female.

Families

There exists a variety of familial structures.
Family dynamics may undergo transformations as time elapses.

Each individual possesses distinct qualities and abilities to offer. Family members ensure the wellbeing of one another. Families adhere to a set of guidelines in order to foster harmonious coexistence. Despite residing in disparate locations, individuals within a family can maintain their familial bond.

Personal skills

All individuals, including children, possess inherent rights. Individuals engage in various modes of communication. It is considered acceptable to seek assistance. Commence integrating the process of making informed choices within the confines of one's domestic setting. Every decision carries with it both advantageous and disadvantageous outcomes.

Practice assertiveness.

Hone one's negotiation abilities in order to achieve resolution in problematic situations or conflicts. The assistance they require

This is the phase in which your children possess a willingness to accept and internalize all that you communicate. Therefore, do not squander this valuable chance to establish yourself as their primary authoritative figure. Should you decline to provide it, they will invariably seek it from alternative sources such as acquaintances and various forms of media.

There exists a substantial disparity between the level of knowledge that a child of 5 years old necessitates compared to that of an 8-year-old. As they advance in age, it becomes imperative to provide them with more intricate explanations and reiterate information with greater frequency.

Make an effort to respond to their inquiries with utmost honesty and neutrality. Inquire of them, "What are your thoughts?" - this allows for discerning their existing knowledge and desired knowledge.

Ensure that you provide them with sufficient information to prevent erroneous inferences, such as if you were to state that procreation occurs when a man and woman sleep together, they may mistakenly interpret this as mere physical proximity rather than sexual intercourse.

Ensure that they have comprehended the information provided and ascertain if any additional inquiries are present. Certain children may not pose queries, necessitating your initiative to initiate the discourse.

One can accomplish this by actively seeking everyday situations that offer opportunities for initiating a conversation, such as encountering a pregnant woman, observing a couple engaged in an affectionate act on television, or coming across menstrual products in a restroom. Additionally, you may consider purchasing literature on sexual education to engage in joint reading.

At this stage of development, it is crucial to engage in dialogue regarding the safe navigation of online environments, even if your child is not yet ready to independently access the internet for a few more years.

Implement regulations surrounding interactions with unfamiliar individuals and the sharing of digital imagery, alongside guidelines for addressing situations in which your child encounters content that elicits discomfort.

Thornhill observes that there is no requirement for taking preemptive action. Provide a comprehensive explanation of pornography to children, ensuring their readiness to potentially come across such material.

Convey in a composed manner that such websites are dedicated to adult-oriented content, while emphasizing that it is crucial to highlight their exclusivity for individuals of a mature age.

At this stage of development, it is appropriate to engage in open and direct conversations with children regarding the subject of sexual abuse. Children must be made aware of this regrettable reality, both for their own benefit and that of a peer who may be subjected to abuse.

The level of detail in this discussion is contingent upon your child. Commence by focusing on fundamental principles, such as emphasizing the importance of obtaining consent before physical contact, subsequently readdressing the topic at a later juncture to assess comprehension and ascertain emotional well-being.

In the event that your child becomes upset, it may be advisable to defer discussing this matter until they reach a more appropriate age.

At this juncture, it may be appropriate to elucidate the explicit dynamics of human reproduction to children. There is nothing amiss with presenting this information sooner if your child appears prepared for it, or deferring it slightly if you believe they will not grasp it.

For the sake of facilitating this discourse, I shall propose the inclusion of a well-crafted literary work that specifically addresses the multitude of inquiries your child may have.

Discussing the subject of sexual matters can be closely intertwined with another essential subject matter: the onset of puberty. When children reach approximately six years of age, it is appropriate to engage them in a straightforward conversation regarding the physiological transformations that occur throughout our developmental journey.

For instance, one could juxtapose images capturing their early years with present-day appearances as a means of illustration. Delay discussing the intricacies of puberty until the commencement of your child's or her peers' actual encounter with this phase. Alternatively, "Otherwise, it will give the impression that you are referring to a celestial body unknown to human experience."

Pubertal onset typically occurs in girls between the ages of nine and eleven. For these individuals, a significant signal that this transition is occurring is the emergence of mammary gland buds, a process that typically commences prior to reaching the age of 10.

Menstruation typically occurs at a later stage, usually around the age of 12, although it is not uncommon for it to commence earlier. Male children typically initiate puberty around the age of 10, marked by the development of pubic hair as the initial identifiable indication.

When engaging in a conversation about puberty, it is advisable to provide your child with a reputable publication that elucidates the finer details of this natural process. This resource should cover various technical aspects of puberty, including the distinctions between testosterone and estrogen, the mechanisms underlying changes in bodily features such as hair growth, genital development, and alterations in the vocal range.

To facilitate a more comprehensive discussion. It is not merely a matter of girls receiving one lesson while boys receive another. It is imperative that children acquire knowledge not just about their own bodies but also about the intricacies of the human form in general.

While the intricacies of puberty may be best discussed in a singular conversation, the ramifications of this transformative phase necessitate an ongoing dialogue.

Children of this developmental stage also require a deeper understanding of the breadth of gender expression. If you happen to have avoided delving into this topic, it is essential to acquire knowledge beforehand. Thornhill proposes initiating the dialogue by highlighting the fact that one cannot ascertain an individual's gender solely by examining their genitalia.

www.ingramcontent.com/pod-product-compliance
Lightning Source LLC
Chambersburg PA
CBHW050026130526
44590CB00042B/1967